# SING NO SAD SONGS

*Dedication*

For Chris, Susannah, Benjamin
and Rebecca

**Also by Sandra Arnold**

*A Distraction of Opposites*
*Tomorrow's Empire*

# SING NO SAD SONGS

## LOSING A DAUGHTER TO CANCER

## Sandra Arnold

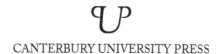

CANTERBURY UNIVERSITY PRESS

Published with the support of Creative New Zealand.

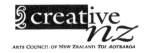

This book began life as Sandra Arnold's thesis for a PhD in
Creative Writing at Central Queensland University.
The exegesis or critical analysis that formed part of that
submission can be found online at
www.cup.canterbury.ac.nz.

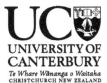

**UNIVERSITY OF
CANTERBURY**
*Te Whare Wānanga o Waitaha*
CHRISTCHURCH NEW ZEALAND

First published in 2011 by
CANTERBURY UNIVERSITY PRESS
University of Canterbury
Private Bag 4800, Christchurch
NEW ZEALAND
www.cup.canterbury.ac.nz

ISBN 978-1-927145-06-7

A catalogue record for this book is available from the
National Library of New Zealand.

Cover painting by Rebecca Arnold
Cover and page design and layout by Quentin Wilson, Christchurch

Printed by PrintStop Ltd, Wellington, New Zealand

# CONTENTS

# ACKNOWLEDGEMENTS

This book, together with an exegesis on parental bereavement, formed my PhD project and I wish to acknowledge Central Queensland University for the support I received during my candidature. I am also grateful to Associate Professor Wally Woods and Dr Lynda Hawryluk for their invaluable help and critical feedback. A short extract from the book has previously appeared in *TEXT* vol. 14 (2), Special Issue 7, October 2010, and I thank the journal's editors, Professor Jen Webb, Associate Professor Nigel Krauth and Professor Donna Brien.

My deep appreciation to Canterbury University Press's Publisher, Rachel Scott, for her enthusiasm for the manuscript and her efficiency and professionalism in guiding it into the world. Thanks to Quentin Wilson for his sensitive and thoughtful approach to Rebecca's painting in the beautiful cover design. The story of how Rebecca came to do the painting is told in the book. Thanks also to Barry Brailsford for permission to quote his poem, 'Piwakawaka'. Thanks to my dear friends John Allison, Jim Norcliffe, Helen Maidment and Marj Hay for permission to include extracts of their letters. Some names in this book have been changed or omitted to protect the privacy of the individuals concerned.

A huge debt of gratitude goes to my family – Chris, Susannah and Benjamin – for their love and encouragement during the writing of this book. Finally, I acknowledge our beautiful daughter Rebecca, from whom I learnt so much in the 23 years I was privileged to have her in my life.

# FOREWORD

Five years ago I was driving back from Akaroa. A beautiful afternoon, sun shining on bare Canterbury hills. I switched on National Radio and there was a story. Often I dislike the stories: sometimes the voice sounds artificial and strained, sometimes the story feels banal and uninspired. But this story took me by the throat. Two people were travelling in a foreign place, remembering the death of their daughter. It was a dry desert place. They camp on a beach, find a stone with the daughter's initials etched in limpets, watch a turtle struggle across the sand to lay her eggs.

I had pulled over and stopped the car long before that final scene, caught by the power of the words and the overwhelming evocation of grief. It was not until the story had ended that I learned that the author was in fact a friend: Sandra Arnold. In that instant she became someone other than the person with whom I shared coffee and the occasional dinner: she became a mother in the lineage of all those noble and courageous grieving mothers reverenced in art and literature. Someone worthy of profound respect.

Now I have read the context for that story in this book, which recounts the death of a daughter – beautiful, strong, gifted – in words so pure and powerful, so utterly truthful that I am overwhelmed once more.

I am not a fan of those disease-of-the-week TV specials, those slick hospital dramas with their neat conclusions and swelling violins. The very word 'grief' is tossed about, applied to everything from sadness at the loss of a building or a city, to the deaths of millions. It has become in modern parlance a 'process', with predictable therapeutic stages.

This book reclaims the word. It lets in laughter, and delight in a life lived impulsively;

it acknowledges moments of bleak failure and despair; it recounts death without recourse to the conventional reassurance of religion; it offers the gentle comfort of horses and lets the cat in to sit on the sick bed.

It is a brave and wonderful book about death, pain and love.

Fiona Farrell

# INTRODUCTION

*Stray birds of autumn come to my window to sing and fly away.*
*And yellow leaves of autumn, which have no songs,*
*flutter and fall there with a sigh.*
(Tagore, 1916)

On 6 April 2002 my youngest daughter Rebecca died of a rare appendix cancer, at the age of 23. For a whole year afterwards I couldn't say her name and the word 'died' in the same breath. Though I am a writer and a teacher of writing, I had no words to describe this cataclysmic event in the life of my family. I could no longer read novels, listen to music, or watch films. I stopped dreaming. It hurt to breathe. It hurt to be inside my skin. I woke at night with my heart beating hard against my ribs. Large gatherings of people with their noisy laughter and banal chatter suffocated me.

The silence of my own home, the green beauty of my garden, the warm breaths of my cats and dog and goat and horses, the quiet paddocks, the river walks and the mountains provided no refuge. They were all empty spaces that reverberated with Rebecca's absence. This new territory was so bleached of colour, so arid and alien, so lacking in anything recognisable that I had no language to negotiate my way through it. And I could form no response to comments such as, 'Gosh, you're coping so well. I don't know how you do it. Now if this had happened to *my* child ...'

I turned to books on grieving to see if the words of others who'd travelled this road before me could help identify some landmarks. On the shelves of bookshops and libraries I found row upon row of books about infant death, child death, sudden violent teenage death and adult death, but there was almost nothing on the death of a young adult child from cancer. As I worked my way through academic literature, books by grief counsellors, psychologists, clergymen and bereaved parents, I found the reason for this dearth of information: the incidence of cancer in the 18- to 25-year-old age group is extremely rare.

In the years since Rebecca's death, after all my reading and discussion with other bereaved parents, I have come to understand that the experience of grief is different for each individual. Listening to or reading about the stories of others can help us recognise landmarks in unfamiliar territory. However, as Arthur Frank says in *The Wounded Storyteller*, 'People tell stories … not to provide a map that can guide others – each must create his own – but rather to witness the experience of reconstructing one's own map' (1995, p. 17).

This book is the map I have constructed for myself. It is not my husband's map, or our elder daughter's, or our son's. The ways in which they were affected by Rebecca's dying and death are integral to our family story, but in this book they are seen through the lens of my own perspective. Nor did I want Rebecca to be defined by her suffering and death. She was a vibrant, multi-talented young woman and her life, as well as her death, has a context.

Six years before she was diagnosed with cancer, Rebecca, my husband, Chris, and I travelled to Brazil to live and work for one year. There, Rebecca blossomed from a shy, horse-obsessed 16-year-old into a confident young woman as she responded to the foreign environment we lived in and was nurtured and loved by the people around her. Those same people, who adopted us into their extended families when we lived amongst them, continued to support us when Rebecca was dying, and after she died. They still talk about her today as naturally as breathing. Unlike many in our Anglo-Saxon society, they do not shy away at the sound of her name.

New Zealand, where we live, is a beautiful, green and fertile land, but after Rebecca's death Chris and I needed to leave it for a while. A desert country seemed the place that best reflected our inner landscape and so we were drawn to Oman in the Arabian Gulf. We would immerse ourselves in the culture of this alien land that held no memories of the life we'd known.

On our way to work in Oman for a year, we stayed briefly in England, the country of our birth, and with my brother I returned to the scenes of my childhood. This bridge to the past connected me to the present and showed me possibilities for the future. The year in Oman allowed healing to continue in circumstances we could never have imagined. At the end of the year, our journey home to New Zealand took us back to Brazil. There, we were able to look into the shadows of the past while we were embraced once again by the people who loved us and who had loved Rebecca. By the time we returned to New Zealand we were ready to face the future.

# PROLOGUE

**Winter, 2000**

For six weeks rain dripped from a sullen sky. The fords were all flooded, cutting off our access to the roads that would take us from Greendale to Christchurch. The one road remaining open added an extra 30 minutes to the daily hour-long trip. Chris and I had flu and the only one of us enjoying the saturated landscape was Rebecca, who declared it 'cool' to ride her horse through the flooded fords to see how deep they were. Trucks and cars waited on either side to see how far up the horse's legs the water would go before deciding whether they would chance the crossing.

During the transition from winter to spring, Chris's mother died after a stroke, at the age of 92. Her funeral was simple with just the family and the one friend, another English woman, she had made in New Zealand. Most of her friends in England were already dead. Chris, Susannah, Benjamin and Rebecca talked about her life, and how special Momma and Poppa had been to them since coming to New Zealand 15 years ago to live with us. In the background, Poppa's voice sang his favourite songs. A few months after he died, Momma said she wished she could hear his voice again. Benjamin searched in the attic and found the old tapes on which Poppa had recorded himself singing in England, where he used to be in a male voice choir. Benjamin transferred the songs onto a CD and told Momma he had a surprise for her. When she heard the familiar music and Poppa's voice, tears of happiness streamed down her face.

At the funeral, when Poppa's voice finished singing, we all sat for a moment thinking about their long life in England, filled with friends and adventures; the death of their first baby; their happiness when Chris was born 12 years later, when they'd given up all hope of having a child; their decision to uproot themselves from England and join us in New Zealand. After 60 years of marriage it was hard for Momma to bear the eight-year separation Poppa's death had brought, but she bore it far more stoically than I thought I'd be able to under the same circumstances.

For her 90th birthday we'd taken her for a helicopter ride. She emerged from the helicopter with her three grandchildren and a huge smile on her face. Susannah told her that her next birthday present would be a bungee jump. She laughed and laughed. Then she told us matter-of-factly that she hoped she wouldn't be in this world on her next birthday. She'd enjoyed her life, but it had gone on far too long. Her only regret was that she didn't have a great-grandchild. This wish came true two years later to her utter delight, when Benjamin and Dee announced Dee's pregnancy. However, she got progressively frailer after a series of strokes and missed the birth of her first great-grandchild by six weeks.

The sun came back, our health returned, snowdrops and bluebells and daffodils pushed through the sodden earth. Apple and plum and cherry blossom frothed the trees. Thrushes, blackbirds and silver-eyes built their nests. Lambs filled the paddocks. In the middle of such fecundity, four weeks before his time, our family's new baby was born. Elliot lay in his incubator like a tiny white frog attached to wires and drips and it was two weeks before Benjamin and Dee could take him home.

It made my heart thump to watch Benjamin's tenderness with his new son. It made me cry to inhale his newborn smell and touch the silky folds of skin that hung off his minuscule limbs like an oversized suit. As he grew to fit his skin we scanned his face for inherited characteristics. His mother's mouth. His father's eyes. His grandfather's stubbornness. I remembered when Momma and Poppa, and later my parents, visited us in the USA a few months after Susannah was born. Only now did I comprehend their helpless devotion to the newest offspring and their barely-held-in-check desire to offload their opinions about the 'right' way to bring her up. Then this was all repeated when Benjamin was born four years later in England, and Rebecca three and a half years after that, in New Zealand.

In October, after a family dinner to celebrate Susannah's 30th and Benjamin's 26th birthdays, we buried Momma's ashes in our rose garden and planted a yellow freesia rose on top. Elliot slept in his pram while we completed our ceremony.

'Mum, did you see the fantail?' Rebecca asked.

'What fantail?'

'It sat on that tree and watched us the whole time. How come you didn't see it?'

'It's a piwakawaka – a spiritual messenger in Maori tradition,' Susannah said. 'I think the fantail was Momma's way of letting us know she's free.'

'It's just a bird,' I said.

Chris commented that he and I were now the 'older generation'. According to statistics, he said, he'd be next on the list to go. This brought an anguished howl of 'Da-aaad!' from the three kids. And a shiver from me.

**23 October 2001**

**Artist Profile**

Rebecca is 23 years old and lives in North Canterbury with her horses, dogs, cats, chickens and a goat. She has painted all her life and is currently studying for a degree in Art and Design at Christchurch Polytechnic Institute of Technology. She works mostly in acrylics, oil pastels, pencil and charcoal. Her paintings often reflect the vibrant colours of the skies, farmlands and mountains of her environment, and the energy and grace of the horses she has spent much of her life training. Recently she has been experimenting with painting the human form and capturing the enigma of the human spirit.

**6 April 2008**

The sky is that dazzling, cloudless blue of a typical Canterbury autumn day. Sunlight shimmers on the leaves of the pin oak outside my study window, turning them into little red flames. A friend once told me she found where I lived much too quiet. 'Sandra,' she breathed, wide-eyed with dismay, 'I heard a *leaf* falling!'

A truck hurtles down the gravel road, shattering the stillness, sending up clouds of dust. The sheep, grazing in neighbouring paddocks, ignore it. There's a light dusting of snow on the tops of the Alps. No wind yet, but later there'll be gusts, scattering red and gold leaves around my garden. It's the same sort of day as the day Rebecca died.

Chris has taken Rebecca's huntaway, Scrappy, for a walk along the river. This evening, at 9.45, we'll light a candle. Susannah will light hers in Christchurch and Benjamin will light his in Wellington. At 10.10 we'll blow it out. Rebecca slipped out of this world six years ago as easily as she entered it 23 years before that.

I settle into a chair to spend the morning reading a folio of stories and essays Rebecca wrote for her sixth form correspondence school course when we lived in Brazil in 1995. I haven't read these stories since and I need to take a deep breath before I open them now. Some silver sprinkles in the shape of birds and hearts fall out of the file as I take out the sheaf of papers. I didn't know they were in there. They must have fallen from a packet Susannah's friend, Sari, sent me with the cards she made from some of Rebecca's artwork.

The first story I open is called 'Te Amo' (I Love You) and is about a boy whose parents had died in a house fire two years previously. He'd been unable to grieve for them. One day riding on the beach he is overcome with misery and sets his mare free, telling it to return to the forest and live at liberty. When he goes home he sees the mare lying injured on the road. Someone had sent for a humane killer and the boy witnesses the mare being shot. With his grief for the horse, the boy is at last able to release his pent-up tears for his parents. The story ends with him deciding to help the man bury the mare. This assuages his guilt for not attending his parents' funeral:

*She was his responsibility. He would accept her death and help bury her. He would also bury his memories and start a fresh life. The boy kissed his little mare on the nose, a final goodbye, and went to tell the killer he was ready.*

The second story is about three young people on the run for killing the king's guards. One suggests they try to find Camelot.

*To go back is to die. To go forward at least gives us a chance to live, to have a future. What else is there to do? Wander around in circles until the soldiers come and kill us?*

Is this Rebecca's message? Each anniversary there's been one.

The next story is 'Real Soil is Grey', based on Rebecca's experiences in her first few weeks in Brazil as she embraced an alien way of life. As I read each story, memories untangle themselves from dusty layers. My tears fall onto the paper. I brush the tips of my fingers over the familiar handwriting, carelessly scrawled across the page. There are many crossings-out on the first drafts of these stories. Here and there Rebecca had stopped and pondered about the best way to say something, and started again. The finished drafts were tidier. She cared about the final impression. She wanted to get a good mark and she did. Some of the stories were published in the Correspondence School magazine for the best work that year.

Two days before this sixth anniversary, Chris and I had gone to the wedding of one of his colleagues. The reception was at Mona Vale, a beautiful, old, colonial house and garden by the Avon River, where Susannah had had her wedding reception 11 years earlier. As we drank champagne in the garden, waiting for the bridal party to arrive, I looked up at the balcony where Susannah and her two bridesmaids had posed for photos. There was the space where Rebecca had stood, smiling, elegant in her long, blue dress. In Brazil she'd been thrilled to hear of her sister's engagement to Mark and their invitation to her to be a bridesmaid, but dismayed when she learned she'd have to wear a dress. 'What's wrong with jeans?' she asked, perplexed with my firm no.

Back in New Zealand, in the dress shop, she hitched the slim-fitting, blue dress above her knees and strode in her thick, woollen socks and riding boots across the floor to the mirror. 'Well, how on earth am I meant to walk in this?' she complained, as we all burst out laughing. But in the porch of the church she asked me to check if her shoulders were back, if she was standing straight, if her walk was ladylike enough. She was concentrating so hard on ladylike that she forgot to hand over Susannah's bouquet to the other bridesmaid, Tanya, who had to prise it from her white-knuckled fingers. At the reception friends asked me tentatively where Rebecca was. Wasn't she going to be a bridesmaid?

'That's her.'

'You're joking!'

'No.'

'Good God!'

They blinked at her, struggling to match the horse-obsessed, pony-tailed tomboy in grubby jeans, who jumped over gates rather than slow down long enough to open them, with this gorgeous 18-year-old, graciously serving wedding cake.

Another bridesmaid now moved into the space Rebecca had briefly occupied 11 years ago. The guests milled about the lawns with their glasses of champagne. Japanese tourists took photos before being discreetly moved on by the Mona Vale staff. A punt, with a young couple on board, floated dreamily down the Avon in the dying sunlight.

A few weeks before this anniversary I dreamt I was watching a Maori mother holding the ashes of her son in her hand. The tips of the ashes were glowing, as if on fire. *This is all she has*, I thought. In the dream, a group of other mothers gathered around telling me of the deaths of their children. I listened and ached for them, in the same way I ache, deep in my belly, every time I hear of a child's death.

A friend once told me that when her baby died, she thought the world would stop spinning on its axis. It was incomprehensible, she said, when she heard of the next cot death. And the next. Then the next. Soon, the world seemed to be full of cot deaths, in the same way that when we were pregnant it was full of babies.

On the first anniversary of Rebecca's death I stood at my study window looking at the fog shrouding the Southern Alps and drifting low over the paddocks. Rebecca used to say she disliked seeing the mountains obscured by fog because she felt disorientated. When she could see the mountains she knew she was home. I turned away from the window and opened the front door. *It's gone on too long*, I thought. *I want her back*. A fantail flew into the living room, perched on a ceiling beam then flew back out into the garden. It circled around Chris's head and disappeared into the trees. We were both moved to tears by this visit of the piwakawaka. But 'forever' without Rebecca lay far beyond our ability to comprehend.

The shape and size of 'forever' started to become clearer a few months after the second anniversary, by which time we'd returned to New Zealand from a year in Oman. I was driving home from Darfield, our nearest town. As I drove over a ford and round the corner I looked in my rear-view mirror and saw the road and trees rapidly receding into the distance. I understood in that moment that as our family moved further into the future, Rebecca would be left further behind. Her life with us and with her friends, her hopes and dreams and plans, were already frozen in the past. Nothing new would be added to her strand of our family story.

As the years passed, the links that bound her to us would gradually fade and disappear. First her favourite horse died. Then the abandoned newborn goat she'd brought home and fed every two hours throughout the first few nights died at the age of nine. Most recently, one of her adored Siamese cats, Song, died, aged 16. One day Chris noticed that Song couldn't walk properly. That night we left her in her bed by the fire. Chris got up to see if she was still alive. She was. Just. Next morning the vet came out. We lifted Song onto Chris's lap. The vet injected her. She listened to her heart with her stethoscope and said, 'She's gone.' We let her sister, Sing, sniff her. I wrapped Song in a soft fleece scarf that Rebecca had worn when all her hair fell out after chemo and we buried her near the rowan tree under which Rebecca's ashes lie.

For months afterwards Sing paced around the house calling or just staring at the hall door crying. She got worse. The noise was harsh and loud. In desperation we brought the huntaway, Scrappy, into the house to keep her company. Rebecca had brought him home 10 years before, aged six months, to help her round up sheep on Kevin's farm. Unaccustomed to being in the house he was ecstatic in his new role as cat comforter and was happy to let Sing snuggle up under his belly. Rebecca's horse, Red, now living with Mark's sister, Melanie, was 24. How long would we have these three? When they died that would be our last link with Rebecca's animals.

A few months after Rebecca died I noticed people avoided mentioning her name, or they changed the subject when I spoke about her. A few friends had stopped visiting or ringing when the cancer was diagnosed. Others vanished after her death. As months and then years went by, it was obvious they'd never make contact. How easy it would be, I realised, for Rebecca to be erased.

Soon after our return from Oman we discussed with Susannah and Benjamin whether or not we should clear Rebecca's room. They agreed it was time. She wouldn't have wanted us to create a shrine. So we took down the posters of horses and film stars, and drawings and horse ribbons, and the calendar with riding events scribbled over various dates. We packed her clothes and paints and easel in boxes and put them in the attic. We gave away all her *Horse and Pony* magazines and repainted the walls. Giving away her horse-riding gear proved too hard and it stays in the barn, gathering dust. The old barn is on its last legs. When we build a new one I'll give the saddles and bridles and blankets to the Riding for the Disabled School. It was through volunteering there from the age of 11 that Rebecca's passion for horses grew.

As I took the notices and postcards, get-well cards and photos off the wallboard, I found a scrap of paper tucked under a little brass horseshoe. Scribbled on the paper in Rebecca's handwriting was *13th February, 2002*. It was the date scheduled for the operation that would try to reverse the detested ileostomy. But the horseshoe must have run out of luck.

Two years after we returned to New Zealand from Brazil, one year after we started living in our beautiful cottage in the country, four years before she died, Rebecca painted a picture of a witch with long, blonde hair, big boobs and a broomstick. She gave it to me for Christmas. In the witch's hand is a bright gold flash of magic, shaped like a spiderweb. Four years later, Susannah gave me a witchy broomstick for my birthday. I walked down our long drive to collect the post, with Susannah calling that I should fly down on the new broomstick. When I reached the postbox there was a beautiful spiderweb, strung between the postbox and a rosebush. It flashed gold in the sunlight.

I sold the last of the horses when we came back from Oman and the paddocks stood empty and silent. Chris thought we should grow trees there, but I couldn't stand the lack of movement and Susannah and I went out and bought three alpacas. Knowing nothing much about alpacas except that we liked to spin their fleece, Susannah and I started going to workshops to learn as much as we could. One of these was a neo-natal workshop. We had to practise delivering dead cria from an artificial uterus. Oh, the cold, lifeless little forms. Susannah touched my arm and asked if I was okay. I nodded, but I wasn't sure. An old man opposite me had tears in his eyes. The girl running the workshop noticed our forlorn expressions and said, 'You can't hurt these little guys. But what you learn today may help save a live cria and its mother.' That made me feel a little better.

The day Susannah gave me the broomstick she helped me scoop up the alpaca poo and dig it into the flowerbeds. We sat on the barrels Rebecca had placed under the pine trees so I could watch her training the horses. Susannah said that when she saw her mother-in-law and her sister together she felt desolate as she realised she would never grow old with her own sister like that. Rebecca had always been her baby sister, but the seven year age gap had been narrowing as Rebecca entered her twenties.

'We could've been companions,' she said. 'She was so laidback once she got over her teenage years.'

Rebecca was laidback as a baby too. On the rare occasions she cried there were no tears. When she was nine months old, I took her to the doctor to find out why it was she never cried tears. He looked at me and raised one eyebrow. I was worried that my baby *didn't* cry? I should just go home and be thankful.

She did cry at age six, when her mouse died. She buried it in the garden with two iceblock sticks attached in the shape of a cross to mark the grave. Then dug it up several times over the next few weeks to see how the decomposition was going. She didn't cry when she fell and skinned her knees, which she did often, as she liked pretending she was a horse that jumped over barriers she built in the garden. She didn't cry when her real horse kicked her 15-year-old head and she needed stitches, nor five years later, when her forehead was split open by an ice hockey stick at the start of a game.

Soon after the family moved from Christchurch to Greendale, in North Canterbury, a letter arrived from David in Brazil to tell us that the mare and foal we'd bought from him for Rebecca's 17th birthday had died:

*The news of Cristiane and Beija-Flor isn't so good. We traded Cristy to a neighbour soon after you left for a very beautiful and tame mare named Andorinha (Swallow). Cristy was fine until the birth of her colt during which they both died. Then Beija-Flor, still with us, did not respond to the treatment for his anaemia, got thinner and thinner and ended up dying last month.*

We didn't know how we were going to break this news to Rebecca. Chris went out and bought her a copy of *Shy Boy*, the original horse-whisperer, Monty Roberts' book. He gave it to her and said we'd had a letter from David.

Rebecca looked at us.

'They're dead aren't they?'

We nodded, unnerved.

She disappeared into her room for a couple of hours and when she emerged, dry-eyed, she said she was glad they were dead as they would have had a horrible life in Brazil.

At a family dinner celebrating Chris's birthday, just a couple of weeks before her cancer was diagnosed, she said she wouldn't cry when her Siamese cats Sing and Song died, but she would probably commit suicide.

'That's not funny! You shouldn't joke about that!'

'I'm not joking. I couldn't live without my cats. How long do cats live anyway?'

'Seventeen to 20 years.'

'So another eight years, then? I'll be 30! My God! Thirty! I don't want to be that old!'

'You won't have much choice unless you cark it before then!' retorted Benjamin.

'Well, I'm not bothered. I know I won't live till I'm 30.'

Howls of protest from Susannah. 'D'ya mind! *I'm* 30!'

A snort from Benjamin. 'You do talk rubbish at times.'

She didn't cry in the recovery room 11 months later when the surgeon told her he was very sorry, but he hadn't been able to reverse the ileostomy as the tissue was now full of cancer. Her face was stony and she wouldn't look at him. She told me she hated him for doing the ileostomy in the first place, without her permission.

'There was no time to ask you. It was an emergency operation. Your appendix burst. He did it to save your life.'

'I'd rather have died.'

Two weeks before she died she looked at photos in her album. She said, 'If I could have only one wish it would be just to be normal again.'

I didn't see her tears then, but later I found a pile of wet tissues by the chair. The album was open at the photo of Rebecca and her best friend, Natasha, shovelling up horse poo in the paddocks, the Southern Alps sparkling under a bright blue sky. The girls were 19. We'd been back in New Zealand one year, and had moved to Greendale just a few weeks previously. On the day I took the photo we were pretending we were on holiday.

Rebecca said, 'Do you think the owner of this place would let us have it another weekend?'

'Probably not,' I grinned. 'If you lived here, would you let anyone else have it?'

And we almost hugged ourselves for having found this beautiful cottage, the tree-filled garden with the swimming pool, the paddocks and the pet sheep. When Rebecca and Natasha brought their horses from the paddock they rented in town and installed them in our own paddocks, their faces could barely contain the width of their smiles.

Since childhood, all Rebecca's drawings and paintings had been of farms and animals. When she was six, she gave me a crayoned picture of a wiggly oval shape covered in coloured spikes.

'What is it?'

'A sheep.'

'And what are these spikes?'

'They're his sparkles.'

'Sparkles?'

'Yes, he's so happy he's sparkling!'

The day I took the photograph of Rebecca and Natasha in the paddock, they were so happy they were sparkling.

# ONE

# Brazil

**1995**

The first blast of scorching air reminded us that none of the clothes we'd brought from New Zealand were going to be suitable for Brazil. Our hotel in Rio de Janeiro was close to the sea. The beach, however, was covered with litter and tiny paper boats with the remains of candles, all that was left of the previous night's celebrations of the *Festa de Iemanja*, the Goddess of the Sea. Further up the beach there'd been a New Year's Eve concert with Rod Stewart.

'What a rubbish dump,' Rebecca grumbled, losing no opportunity to let us know she was here against her will. What on earth made us think she'd enjoy living in a rubbish dump for a year when she was happy back in New Zealand with her friends, training her horse for the Springston Trophy? She could've stayed with Susannah, hadn't we thought of that? And no, of course Susannah wouldn't have minded looking after her for a year. And no, she didn't want to give it time. She didn't like it here. It was too hot, too dirty, too … too … too … *everything*. So could we please just send her home?

Next day we flew in a small plane to Uberaba from where we were supposed to continue our flight to Uberlândia. Without warning, everybody got off the plane. A passenger who spoke English told us that the plane's computer wasn't working. Suddenly everyone turned round and got back on the plane. Apparently, the computer was now operational. By this time, Rebecca was shaking. She liked telling people there were only two things she was afraid of – earthquakes and migraines. Looking at her white face, I wondered if she'd now add flying to that list.

We didn't feel too confident about the plane either, but it managed to make the journey. At Uberaba we were told that the airport in Uberlândia was closed because of bad weather, so we'd be taken there by taxi. The taxi driver drove with his foot flat on the accelerator, overtaking enormous trucks and hurtling straight at oncoming traffic. We closed our eyes. An hour later, to our utter astonishment, we arrived in Uberlândia in one piece.

Camacho and his father were there to meet us and enfolded us in delighted embraces. To Rebecca's horror they hugged and kissed her. I'd warned her that this was the Brazilian way of greeting, but she didn't believe it until she was on the receiving end. We'd asked Camacho to book us into a hotel, but this went against the tenets of Brazilian hospitality, and he told us we were to be his guests in his house for a few days and he'd go apartment hunting with us. Camacho and Stela's two daughters, Tatiana, six, and Gabriella, 10, still retained their New Zealand accents from their four years in Christchurch where Chris had supervised Camacho's PhD.

We spent the next few days looking at a variety of apartments and houses with Camacho. All the houses had high walls with broken glass embedded along the top, heavily locked iron gates and barred windows.

'Is because of the high crime rate,' explained Camacho. 'Is not like in New Zealand.'

Rebecca shot us an *I told you didn't I?* look.

The windows were small with frosted glass.

'Is for the security, but also for the sun, to keep out.'

Plastic bottles, cigarette packets and paper bags lay in piles in the streets and empty sections and graffiti covered every flat surface. Weeds grew out of cracks in the cobbled pavements and the potholes in the roads. Camacho warned us to be careful where we walked and brought his palms up to shoulder height. 'The city council it have no money to maintain.'

There was no system of renting furnished houses. 'The people they no trust tenants to take care. Is not like in New Zealand.' He made several phone calls and on the third day he located a woman he knew who owned and rented out furnished apartments in an apartment-hotel in the city centre. A swimming pool, gym and sauna occupied the roof, and tennis and badminton courts the top floor. We moved in that evening.

After moving in we spent most of our time getting to grips with bureaucracy and the Brazilian way of doing things. The shops were not easily identifiable because of all the bars and grilles over them, but after a few weeks we began to find life more manageable. However, Rebecca was shocked by the mangy dogs she saw everywhere. She patted one and it tried to follow her. We saw an injured kitten lying in the middle of the road. Nobody stopped to help. It flipped over to the gutter and crawled under a car. Rebecca was distraught that we told her to leave it. There was nowhere to take it for help. Camacho told her that when he was living in New Zealand he couldn't believe it when he saw all the traffic come to a halt on Memorial Avenue to let a duck and her ducklings cross the road. 'If that happen here,' he said, 'you see feathers everywhere, isn't it?'

The Brazilian government was trying to keep inflation under control and it was running at 3 per cent per month as opposed to the 700 per cent a month the previous year. The country had enormous mineral wealth and natural resources, Camacho said, but the profits went into the hands of a few. Taxes were high, but went to support the bureaucracy in the capital city of Brasilia. There was no money to pay for basic facilities such as a good public health and education system. Camacho said that when his department needed a new photocopier they all clubbed together and bought one. He also told us that he had painted the office that Chris was going to use. 'I felt ashamed,' he said, 'to put you in there the way it was.'

The city was crowded with young people who'd come to take their university entrance exams. One evening we were sitting at a roadside café eating ice creams. The pavements were crowded with teenagers laughing and dancing. There was a display of *capoeira* near our table. Recognising we were foreigners, a young man who spoke English explained it was a traditional form of martial art, developed when Brazil had slaves. They weren't allowed to fight, so they disguised their movements as dancing. The traffic jammed up in the street and drivers kept their hands on their horns to add to the general racket of the singing and dancing and rock bands. Those who lost patience simply turned around and went the wrong way down one-way streets.

Nobody seemed to take much notice of traffic signals and we didn't see anyone wearing a bike helmet, even on a motorbike. If drivers couldn't find a parking place they parked on the pavements. Negotiating these was fraught with danger as they were full of parked cars, potholes and demolition gangs throwing bricks around. It was easier to walk in the roads except there were very few pedestrian crossings and it wasn't obvious when to cross. One day we saw the front wheels of a truck entirely engulfed in a hole in the road. Camacho said it was a council truck, so it deserved to fall in as the council was responsible for the roads.

We visited the English Language School in Araguarí where I was going to start teaching the following month. It belonged to Sebastião and Marilia, friends of Camacho.

I spotted a large lizard parked in a corner of the bathroom. Rebecca said, 'Oh! *Cool*!' I said, 'AAARRGH!' Marilia said it kept down the mosquitoes.

In the evening they took us to a restaurant set in a park full of lush trees and bushes. Enormous yellow butterflies fluttered in the foliage over the windows. A singer began playing his guitar and crooned into the microphone. His voice was warm, melted honey. Chris stopped eating and listened to him, entranced. He scribbled a note in English, 'Your singing is superb!' Calvino, the singer, read the note and waved at us, smiling broadly.

Marilia asked Rebecca how she was settling in. Rebecca glanced at us, coughed politely and murmured that she was missing her cats, her horse, and her brother and sister.

'Your brother and sister?' Chris and I chorused. 'Would you like to put that in writing so we can frame it?'

She pretended she hadn't heard. Sebastião told her he and Camacho were going to arrange for her to go to classes at a local high school so she could meet other teenagers, and they were also going to arrange private lessons with a Portuguese teacher for all of us. Rebecca paled. What she wanted was to go back to New Zealand, though I was impressed with her restraint in not saying this to Marilia. She missed the open spaces and freedom, and the sight of people living in cardboard boxes on the pavement reminded her constantly that she was in a foreign environment that she'd never wanted to come to in the first place. She wrote a postcard to Susannah:

> Hi, how are you?
>     I hope you are really looking after my babies for me! Give them lots of food and cuddles. I really miss you, Ben and Momma and my cats. I hate it here and I want to come home.
>     Love, Rebecca

Over the next few weeks we established a routine. Chris went round the corner to the baker's to buy fresh rolls for breakfast, which we ate with slices of mango, pineapple and guava. Then Chris walked to the university and Rebecca did her sixth form New Zealand Correspondence School work till lunch time. I worked on a new novel. Although lunch, consisting of rice and beans, was the main meal of the day for Brazilians, it was too hot for us to eat anything but fruit. After lunch we went up to the rooftop pool to have a swim while the maid cleaned the apartment. We also swam in the evenings when the temperature dropped from 35 to 25 degrees. One evening two girls about Rebecca's age swam up to her and touched her cheek.

'Your eyes. Beautiful. Very beautiful. You … *muita bonita!*'

Rebecca looked at me, startled. Then blushed and smiled at the girls. 'Er … *obrigada.*'

I turned away to hide my own smile.

From the rooftop we liked watching the way the sun dropped behind a little blue church that looked like a music box, and threw purple shadows over the traffic-clogged city, the sparkling new high-rise apartment buildings and office blocks, to the wastelands of the outer suburbs with their *favelas* of corrugated iron, cardboard and sticks. Then, suddenly it was dark and the city lights came on, obliterating the ugliness we could see by day and creating an illusion of beauty.

We started going to a large supermarket at the mall once a week. There were local shops nearer to our apartment, but the assistants and customers didn't seem to worry about the flies crawling all over the meat and fish. I asked Camacho why they didn't use fly sprays.

'Is bad for health,' he said.

There were stalls along the sides of the roads selling fresh fruit drinks. Rebecca was suspicious of these until Sebastião stopped the car at a stall that sold *ascerola.* The girl put the cherry-like fruit into a blender, strained it, added sugar and water and the result was a divine drink that had the added bonus of weaning Rebecca off Coca-Cola. The girl told Sebastião that she hadn't heard of New Zealand. It was close to Australia, he explained. No, she hadn't heard of Australia either, but she hoped we would have a very happy stay in Brazil.

We stayed at Sebastião's house for the weekend and went to their country club, which was set in parkland surrounded by palm trees. There were several swimming pools, tennis courts, a bar and restaurant and barbecue areas beside cool fountains.

'Because we're not close to a beach, this is where the people who live inland come to rest at weekends,' Sebastião explained.

Marilia's four nephews arrived: Leonardo, Frederiko, Angelo and Evalbe. All tall, tanned, gorgeous teenage boys. Marilia had explained to them that they shouldn't kiss Rebecca as New Zealand teenagers didn't greet like that and she wasn't used to it, so they should just say hi. Marilia turned away to say something to me then looked back and gasped. 'Those boys! Look at them. They're exaggerating it!' They were standing in a line with big grins on their faces and each was kissing Rebecca on both cheeks as she went redder and redder.

Later, I said to her with mock sympathy, 'That must have been embarrassing.'

She shrugged, 'I'll get used to it,' and ran off to join the boys on the hydro slide.

In the evening we went back to the restaurant where we'd first heard Calvino. He was there again and the boys translated some of his lyrics for Rebecca. She listened to this with great interest. They told her he was recording his music at present so we should buy his CD before we left Brazil. After the meal the boys asked us if they could take Rebecca to a local bar where all their friends congregated at the weekends.

'A bar? She's only 16!'

Rebecca's face fell.

'Don't worry,' said Sebastião, 'they'll look after her.'

She told us the next day that they'd danced in the street outside the bar; she'd made lots of friends and she really liked Brazil now. Chris and I looked at each other with raised eyebrows. And breathed a sigh of relief.

Later in the morning we went to Marilia's brother's farm. The soil was red with iron and the contrast between that and the lush green fields was straight out of a paint-by-numbers picture. Mango, banana, guava and lime trees surrounded the farmhouse. Valerio, Marilia's brother, warned us not to walk too near the trees because of the poisonous toads and snakes.

Rebecca's eyes sparkled. '*Snakes*? Cool.'

'No so cool if the snake he on the end of your foot!' laughed Leonardo.

The farmhouse was presently occupied by a manager, but Valerio said he planned to retire from his job as a pilot in about five years' time and live here himself and run cattle. The house was a simple, white, rectangular building with a red-tiled roof. The biggest spiders in the world lurked in star-shaped webs in every corner of the verandah. The smell of pig shit wafted on the hot air into the open kitchen at the back of the house. However, Marilia had brought mountains of food to prepare and a delicious meal appeared, so I closed my eyes to the swarming flies and the spiders waiting for them and tried to ignore the frantic look on Rebecca's face.

Sebastião took us on a tractor ride around the farm to a waterfall. We stood in a wooden cart precariously attached to the tractor, which lurched and bumped over the track. He asked Rebecca if she wanted to drive. Her pained expression cracked under the weight of her delighted smiles. At the end of the track we jumped off and walked a little way to reach the waterfall and swimming hole and stood under the warm, cascading waters of the falls, feeling like Indiana Jones. Later, Angelo brought his horse out for Rebecca to ride. She took off at a gallop. On her return she casually shrugged off their admiration for her riding skills, but she glanced at me and smiled.

As we got ready to leave at the end of the day, all the boys lined up to kiss her again. This time her bright red blush gave way to a pale pink. On the way back to the apartment she said she needed to go shopping for a Brazilian-style bikini.

'I felt like a nun in that black thing I bought in New Zealand!'

Chris told her he didn't know nuns wore swimsuits.


Rebecca's words tumbled over each other in her excitement. On the way to the farm the truck had broken down. A couple of the boys went off to get a tow rope. The others, with Rebecca, sat under the truck to keep out of the blazing sun. '*Sooooooo* cool!'

Magna, Marilia's sister, brought her palms to her shoulders. 'Cool? Under the truck? What kind of girl is this?'

This bewildered acknowledgement that she wasn't a typical girl brought a wide grin from Rebecca. She'd been driving the tractor again – in third gear, she emphasised, and helped to plant corn. They all had an enormous lunch of rice and beans then piled onto the beds to go to sleep for a couple of hours. The boys taught her some Portuguese and Valerio insisted on her using it. She wanted to learn Portuguese now, she said, so she could understand what everyone said.

The experiences of this day, and the resulting turnaround in Rebecca's attitude to Brazil, appeared in fictional form a few months later in an essay for her Correspondence School English course. She called it 'Real Soil is Grey'.

*Later, when they went back to the farmhouse, the boys asked Kara if she would like to help them plant corn in a paddock. The boys started a dirt fight with silver fertiliser. Kara stood back and watched them. She remembered how back in New Zealand she and her friends had mud fights. Just then one of the boys plastered her face with silver fertiliser. Laughing, she grabbed a handful of fertiliser and rubbed it in his face. Suddenly they were all in the middle of a mud fight, laughing and shouting, while the adults sat calmly, drinking beer in the shade of a mango tree, chatting away. What a musical sounding language it is, thought Kara.*

The story finishes with an observation of what 'Kara' had learned in this foreign environment and how good it felt to be befriended there. When the story was printed in the Correspondence School magazine, Marilia asked Rebecca if she could keep a copy. After Rebecca died, Marilia wrote to me saying she'd found the story again and asked if she could use it with her advanced English students. But that was still seven years in the future.

The boys went back to their home towns of Belo Horizonte and São Paulo at the end of the week as the school term was due to start. Rebecca wanted to be fluent in Portuguese before they came back to the farm on their next school holiday. She got out the dictionary and started a notebook of phrases and vocabulary, beginning with the names of everything on the farm. Valerio and his son, Leonardo, told her they travelled from São Paulo every weekend to attend to the farm and they invited Rebecca to go there with them. That was good news for her as she was doing an agriculture course as part of her Correspondence School programme and needed regular access to a farm.

Sebastião brought over a friend's daughter, Anna-Marie, to meet Rebecca. She was a couple of years older than Rebecca, tall and slim with a shaved head that emphasised her fine cheek bones. She told us that it was usual for boys to have their heads shaved when they passed their university entrance exams, but she'd shaved hers just because she felt like it. Rebecca's eyes sparkled. This was her kind of girl. She invited Rebecca to a movie that night with her and her friends. She also invited us all to a barbecue to meet her family the following Sunday.

Rebecca wrote to her brother and sister:

Dear Susannah and Benjamin,

Hi how R U? I really like Brazil now, and I LOVE the farm. I went there last weekend with the boys. I spent 3 days there; the second day was the best! Leonardo was driving the tractor and the rest of us were piled on every spare place on it. We had a mud fight and we came back real dirty. I can't wait to go back to the farm!

How are my baby cats? Give them a huge cuddle from me, I really miss them!!! How is life back in NZ? At the moment it is raining here but it is still very HOT! I don't think I'll ever get used to the temperature!

Tonight I'm going to the movies with Anna-Marie and her friends but the movie probably will be dubbed in Portuguese, but oh well, never mind it's better than staying in this damn apartment!!!

The people here are real nice and friendly and the boys are gorgeous, especially Leonardo!!! It was nice hearing your voice yesterday, I still feel homesick, though I like Brazil now and I'm glad I came, it's hard living here and will take some getting used to. The people make you feel at home (the Brazilian rule is 'there's always room for one more').

Well I've got to go now, Tchau.
Lots of love
Hebecca (that's how my name is pronounced in Portuguese)

Surrounded by slim, well-groomed girls, Rebecca made an effort to lose her puppy fat. This included a self-imposed ban on junk food and she started going to the gym and swimming pool on the rooftop every day. We ate tropical fruit and salads as it was too hot to eat anything else, so Chris and I were also in the process of off-loading several kilos. Rebecca then dumped the clothes she'd brought from New Zealand and started collecting a new wardrobe of stylish Brazilian clothes. She said she'd like to shave her head too, like Anna-Marie.

Julio, an ex-student of Chris's now living in São Paulo state, invited us to visit him and asked Chris to give a seminar at the university in Ilha Solteira. He took us to a Spiritist Church where spiritual healing was taking place and told Rebecca he'd seen spirits himself. Her eyes widened with delight, but he told her this was not the purpose of Spiritism. 'It's more about the philosophy. It's a way of living,' he said. I told him I'd been interested in the topic when I was young as my aunt was a Spiritualist, but I was sceptical of such claims now. He smiled and gave me a book to read on the philosophies of Allan Kardec, the founder of the Spiritist movement in France in the 19th century. 'This might change your mind.'

We visited their country club and in order to get permission to use the swimming pool we had to be medically examined. We donned our swimsuits and went into a room with other examinees while a doctor inspected our toes and hands. Rebecca could barely contain her laughter at my astounded expression.

Julio said small crocodiles and piranha fish lived in the river, but piranhas only attacked if you were bleeding from a cut and the crocs were small so couldn't do much harm. Anna said an anaconda had been seen in the next bay a few days previously. However, the river was full of people swimming, they added, so it would be all right. Anna saw a friend of hers on a jet ski and asked him to take Rebecca for a ride. He zoomed all over the lake with her for about 45 minutes, occasionally making the machine rear up and tip over to each side.

'That's not safe!' I complained to Chris, forcing myself to look in case the jet ski and Rebecca disappeared in a blue flash while I wasn't watching.

'Stop fussing. She'll be fine.'

When Rebecca joined us on the shore she was flushed with excitement. 'That was *awesome*!' she declared.

I put a towel around her shoulders to keep her warm, relieved she was still in one piece, hadn't been swallowed by an anaconda or ripped apart by piranhas.

'You should have a try, Mum!'

I rolled my eyes.

At a farm owned by Julio's friends Artemisia and Alberto, we visited the primitive little wooden house of the farm manager. It had only recently been connected to electricity and the television and fridge looked incongruous on the bare concrete floor with the simple wooden furniture. The manager's wife was making *pamonhas* on the stove outside. We watched her scraping the corn off the cob and boiling it to a pulp with pork fat, then tipping the mixture inside pockets of corn leaves and boiling it again. She gave us one each to try and a large, fat, round cheese to take home with us.

'They don't have much, but they give us what they have,' Rebecca murmured. I rubbed her arm and nodded.

Anna showed Rebecca where she could pick urucum berries. She explained that a red dye could be extracted from the berries that was used by the Indians to paint their faces red. Rebecca was delighted and collected some to use as 'organic material' in her Correspondence School art course. We ended the day by the Paraná, watching storks fly over the river and dragonflies skim the surface of the water. The sun set and washed the sky with orange light.

Next day Anna took us to the zoo, but it was closed. She explained to the manager that we came from a country that had no snakes and that Rebecca really wanted to see one. The manager said in that case he would be happy to give us a personal tour. He showed us boa constrictors, a panther, a leopard, puma, anteaters, tapirs, giant turtles, parrots and monkeys, all animals from the region. He explained that, unfortunately, we'd just missed the feeding of the boa constrictors. Rebecca asked what they ate.

'Live mice,' he said.

She caught my eye and winced.

Before we left for Uberlândia, Julio gave her a present – a little pink clown wrapped up in a pink bow. She was so overwhelmed she could hardly find the words to thank him. This time she had no difficulties with hugging and kissing.

On our return to Uberlândia I started teaching in Araguarí, 30 kilometres away. During the hour-long bus journey I marvelled at the wild and beautiful countryside of the *Cerrado*, while trying to tune in to the loud conversations between passengers at the front of the bus with those at the back. Marilia's father was always there to meet me at the bus station and drive me in his truck to the school, talking to me in Portuguese as if I understood every word and patiently listening to my slow, laborious responses. The two students in my class, Carina and Eliáne, exuberant, talkative young women in their early twenties, were teachers at the school. Carina also studied English Literature at the university. Her dream was to live and work in the USA for a few years. Eliáne had recently married. Her brother had been killed in an accident, she said, so she and her husband lived with her parents as her mother could not get over her son's death.

'I can't imagine a worse thing happening to a parent,' I said.

'Neither can I. When I see my mother – well, that's why I'm afraid to have children,' she replied.

On the bus journey back to Uberlândia each evening I watched spectacular sunsets as sulphurous yellow clouds rolled over an apricot sky shot through with red and gold. Occasionally Rebecca travelled with me and sometimes stayed in Araguarí for the weekends. Her Portuguese was now good enough for her to buy her own bus tickets.

Camacho arranged for her to attend classes at the private high school where he sent his own daughters. She didn't want to go. No one would *talk* to her, and she didn't know enough Portuguese, so how could she talk to *them*? The whole thing was *pointless*. Stela offered to take her and introduce her to the other students. Later Stela rang me and said as soon as they'd got there Rebecca was surrounded by teenagers all wanting to talk to her. Rebecca rang me after school to say she'd been invited to a girl's apartment where a few of them would be doing their homework together, listening to music and dancing. She wouldn't be home till late. The next day she was invited back. The school was, she declared, 'heaps better than in New Zealand' but I suspected that was because it was just another social watering hole where she was, once again, the subject of a great deal of attention.

Stela introduced us to Terezinha, the woman who'd be giving us Portuguese lessons. Terezinha didn't speak any English herself, so that would encourage us to learn Portuguese faster. We'd already picked up quite a bit in three months and the fog of incomprehension was gradually clearing.

Rebecca wrote another note home:

Hi how are you?

I'm great, how's Momma getting on? How are my baby cats? I hear that they are getting fat, well don't over feed them because they are Siamese and they may have a heart attack, don't underfeed them either! Give them lots of attention and play with them a lot too!!! I really miss them. Brazil is great except for the Correspondence work, it's soooooo BORING. I hate it!!! That's all I've got to say, Mum can tell you everything else in great detail!! Say hi to NZ for me.

Tchau,
Rebecca

# TWO

# Dancing to the beat of the band

We were in Porto Seguro, a sea port in Bahia in the north east of Brazil, for *Carnaval*. Pastel-coloured houses, tiny shops, inns and open-air restaurants lined the narrow cobbled streets. Thatched, open-sided *cabanas* on the beaches provided welcome shade from the blazing sun and played music at ear-splitting volume. The tour guide didn't speak any English, but a 16-year-old girl in the group, Gabriella, spoke English fluently so she translated for us, and she and Rebecca spent the whole week together. She introduced us to spicy Bahian food and desserts made of coconut and honey, sold from stalls by women dressed in white lacy dresses and headscarves. Their religion was Candomblé, she said, a kind of voodoo magic that came from the slaves in Africa.

On the beach at night a band played from the top of an enormous truck equipped with giant loudspeakers. I could feel the music vibrating in my bones. Chris and I moved off down the beach to a more tolerable distance while Rebecca stayed near the band with Gabriella and danced all night. All ages, from young children and teenagers to old people, danced under the big, yellow moon. A young father danced with his sleeping baby on his shoulder. A boat came close to shore and the people on the boat started dancing to the music on the beach. Some people threw themselves fully-clothed into the sea.

I watched Rebecca dancing and smiled at her new-found confidence. Brazil was transforming her. She had lost all her puppy fat now and was tanned deep gold. Her hair had lightened several shades with the sun, and with the new style of dressing she'd adopted she no longer looked like the tomboy she'd been just three months before in New Zealand. She was starting to get used to being told by strangers that she was beautiful.

In the *cabana* in front of our hotel we struggled with the menu. A young waiter came over to help.

'I speak a little English,' he said.

He had large hazel eyes, curly brown hair and a beautiful smile. It was soon obvious he knew a lot more than a little English, though he said he'd never been outside Brazil. He told us his name was Fabiano, that he was 21 and a second-year medical student from Belo Horizonte. His friend's uncle owned the *cabana* and he worked here in his vacations. He asked Rebecca about the differences between New Zealand society and Brazil. Rebecca forgot her shyness in her zeal to tell him that in New Zealand people would take an injured animal they found in the street to the vet, and that it was harder to get into vet school than medical school.

His eyes widened. 'You mean animals are more important than people in your country?'

She frowned and told him that in her opinion animals *were* more important than people. He blinked at her and Chris steered the conversation into safer waters by trying out his Portuguese in ordering a fruit juice. Many years later, Fabiano would remind us how touched he was by these stumbling attempts to speak his language.

On our last night in Porto Seguro we went to the *cabana* for dinner. Fabiano wasn't there and one of the other waiters told us he was off duty. We were disappointed as we'd hoped to say goodbye. Within 20 minutes he appeared. The waiter had phoned him to tell him we were there and he hurried over. We exchanged addresses and he said he'd write to us and perhaps come to visit us in Uberlândia.

As we walked back to the hotel over the warm sand, I had the inexplicable feeling that we'd known Fabiano for a long time, and that he would become an important part of our lives in the future. Though Rebecca barely noticed him in Porto Seguro, she did indeed become central to his life, though not till the end of her own life did she appreciate just how special he was.

To her brother and sister she wrote:

Dear Susannah and Benjamin,

Hi how are you? I'm fine. The holiday was lovely. Mum and Dad hated the loud music but I loved it. Mum was right about all the girls swarming in on Benjamin, some of my friends here were asking about the boys in NZ. They said they loved boys with blue eyes and blond hair! In Porto Seguro the sea wasn't warm it was HOT!!! It actually hurt my legs to walk in it! The town was bright and colourful and the people were happy and cheerful and boy did they know how to have a good time!!! Well that's all I've got to say for now. Give my babies lots and lots of cuddles from me and tell them that I really, really, REALLY miss them!!!!!!!!!!!!!!!!!!!!!!. Say hi to momma from me.

    Tchau,

    Lots of love,

    Rebecca

Anna-Marie's family barbecue included all the neighbours in her street, from newborn babies to a man who'd just turned 100. Her mother, a librarian, invited me to give a talk on New Zealand literature to the Uberlândia Writers' Academy. She would arrange for Lilia, a linguistics professor, who spoke both English and Portuguese like a native, as well as her own language, Spanish, to meet me at the *Casa da Cultura* and translate.

Lilia and her American husband, David, came round to the apartment so Lilia and I could meet before the talk. As soon as David set eyes on Rebecca he said, 'Oh, we've got one of those at home too! Betsy. We'll have to introduce you two.'

After the talk at the *Casa da Cultura*, we went to Lilia's house. She'd lived in Brazil since 1982, apart from four years in the States to do her PhD. David was a professor in the Agronomy Department and lectured in Rural Development. Their house, in the oldest part of Uberlândia, was filled with books and beautiful old rural American furniture. They invited us to go to their farm the following Sunday.

At the farm David showed us a bird's nest at the back of the farmhouse and pointed out a flower the bird had stuck in the side of the nest. Laughing, Rebecca took a photograph. In front of the house there was a lake he'd made and filled with fish. The farmhouse had been a summer project for him and his two sons, he said. The two boys had now gone to the USA to finish their education. David was in the process of buying horses and planned to start a horse riding academy for the disabled by the end of the year. One horse was really wild, he said. No one could catch it, let alone ride it. The boy who'd owned it had mistreated it. That boy had recently been killed in an accident and his father now wanted to sell the horse. Rebecca asked to see it.

The farm manager's son, a boy of 13, caught the horse and saddled it and Rebecca mounted. The horse jigged about with its ears laid back, but Rebecca managed to calm it down and took off for a gallop. The horse had an 18-month-old colt which ran after the mare and then three other horses decided to follow, plus the three dogs. We watched Rebecca riding back across the dam with an entourage of animals trailing behind, including a gander, which, David said, always stuck with the horses since his mate had been eaten by something in the lake.

Out on the lake in David's rowing boat I took in the cerulean blue sky, emerald green trees, the red soil, the quaint little wooden farmhouse, the birdsong, the hot earthy smell, and Rebecca on the horse with all the animals in tow. *Hold this moment*, I whispered under my breath.

As we rowed back, the sun began to drop and the horses wandered up to the house and parked themselves on the verandah.

David called to them, 'Go inside, why don't you! Make yourselves at home, sit on the sofa!'

He liked to bring his students out to the farm for the occasional lecture, he said, but first he always had to clear the horses off the verandah.

The house was not habitable as it had wasps' nests inside and it was also full of snakes. David described one day when they were having a picnic by the lake and he looked up and saw a rattlesnake stick its head up and look from side to side just as Betsy was walking towards it. They killed it then searched for the mate because, he said, rattlesnakes are always found in pairs. Rebecca winced. David noticed and said he hated having to kill them.

Walking through the bush we saw a snake about 12 inches long with red, black and white hoops. David said it was a coral snake, deadly poisonous. Rebecca's face lit up – her first wild snake. Lilia, who'd been very reluctant to come into the bush in case she encountered a snake, was horrified. She said her snake phobia sprang from the day she ran into the outside toilet as a child growing up in Panama.

'It was wall-to-wall snake in there,' she said, shuddering. 'I ran screaming back into the house. Stark naked! Right through my parents' dinner party! I've never gotten over it to this day!'

After hearing this I was concentrating so much on what might be wriggling on the ground that I would have walked into a huge wasps' nest hanging off a branch if Chris hadn't pulled me back. I stopped to suck in a deep breath and saw a toucan flying overhead and a scissor-tail land by the lake. Enormous red termite mounds dotted the baked earth. Some were about three feet high with little doorways that had been made by armadillos which used the mounds to live in. That evening Rebecca made three model termite mounds out of red clay and turned them into quirky-looking mice with wide yawns.

A friend of David and Lilia's, Marilena, who taught geography at the university, arrived at the farm with a German who'd been in Brazil for six months doing research on agriculture. She told us he'd caught a snake and put it in the fridge in a plastic bag. She'd then gone to the fridge to take out a bag of sausages for a barbecue. When she got in the car she opened up the plastic bag and saw the frozen snake coiled up at the bottom.

'Imagine if I'd opened it at the barbecue and people thought *that* was *my* contribution!'

We all roared with laughter. Rebecca had tears of delight splashing down her cheeks at the thought of this scene. Marilena asked about our accommodation and when I said we didn't much like living in an apartment in the centre of the city she invited us to share her house when the German and another boarder left in three weeks.

That evening David took Chris and Rebecca to see the outside of Marilena's house.

'You'll love it, Mum,' Rebecca enthused. It was a big house in a large garden on the edge of the city, she said. Chris thought it would be a lot cheaper than the apartment and a lot quieter.

That night we were woken by the usual car alarms screaming and drivers honking their horns maniacally, but this time, in addition to the normal cacophony there was a choir singing somewhere in the street. When they finished a man yelled out in English, 'I looorrrve you Francisca!' then a car roared away. Marilena's house definitely sounded appealing.

Chris suggested we buy the horse and colt on David's farm for Rebecca's 17th birthday, which was coming up next month. She would be able to train them both and sell them at the end of the year. A buyer was coming to look at them and Rebecca chewed her nails down to the quick in anxiety while waiting for his decision. However, he couldn't even catch the mare, let alone ride it. The horse was now hers. She immediately became immersed in selecting a name for the mare and colt out of the several hundred horse names she'd collected over the past few years. She wrote back home:

Dear everyone,

I'll tell you the details about my 2 horses. The mare is a chestnut roan (chestnut base with white hairs sprinkled in). She has a blaze and 2 hind white socks. Her name is Cristiane. Mum nicknamed her Kiss. She is beautiful. From a distance her coat looks a deep rich chestnut (a bit like Mana). Kiss's colt is a bay.

His name is Tempo Troco, which means Time Change. The troco part has a long story. This is it. Leonardo is called Leo for short. In Brazil people stick O on front of names so it's O Leo. What, you may ask has that to do with Troco? Well, one day Mum pointed out a sign that said troco de oleo which means change of oil. Anyway Mum said, 'Look there's your favourite name', meaning O Leo. When I laughed she said, 'Of course I mean Troco'. So from then on Leo was known as Troco. So as I got to name my colt we named him after Leonardo without anyone knowing.

This year I can train two horses. COOL!!!

Well, got to go.

Tchau

Beck

PS When Mum said I galloped off on Kiss she actually means I walked. I have to go very slow with her because she's really psycho.
PPS. How are my babies? Give them huge cuddles from me!!!
PPPS. Here's some Portuguese.

Oi tudo bem? Portuguese é muito dificile, mas eu quero aprende muito logo. Como é meu gatos? Espero elas é bem!!! Como é NZ? Fale oi todas por meu por favour.

Dear Momma,

Hi how are you. I am great, I love Brazil now, but I still miss New Zealand. How are you getting on having to put up with Susannah and Benjamin? How are my cats? I really miss them. Do they sleep on your bed at night? Have you fully recovered from your accident? I hope so. Have you been watching Shortland St? One of my friends has been writing all about it giving me all the details. I miss watching the TV with you. I have made a lot of friends here in Brazil, both in Uberlândia and in Araguari. Well I better go now. Thank you for your letter.

Tchau,

Rebecca

After we bought the horses the deal I made with Rebecca was that as soon as she'd completed her day's study she was free to do whatever she liked and if Chris was around to take her to the farm she could spend the rest of her time with the horses. She had an agricultural project to do so she looked forward to doing it at the weekends when we went to the farm. She continued going to high school two days a week from 1.00pm to 5.30pm and made a lot of friends. She also came with me once a week when I taught in Araguari and met up with her friends there.

Dear Susannah and Benjamin,

G'day, howz it going? I'm marvy. Life is pretty cool over in Brazil. How are my cats? I hope they're 100per cent excellent!!! Tell them I miss them very, very, very, VERY much!!!!!!! Could you make sure that Song has no more bald patches on her? Check Sing too. I've started school here. I've made heaps of friends there. Me, Mum and Dad are taking Portuguese lessons every Monday morning which means I have to get up at 8 o'clock. Can you believe that!! Oh my god.

The Correspondence School really sux!!! I love going to Araguari in the weekends. I have a lot of friends there too. Sometimes I go on Tuesdays or Fridays with Mum when she goes up to teach at Fisk. Well that's all I can think of to say.

Tchau

Beck

Marilena's home, a large, white, two-storey house with a red-tiled roof was set in an enormous garden with trees and flowers. There was a wide verandah downstairs and a balcony upstairs and hammocks slung between the posts of both. Seu Pedro took care of the garden and his sister, Dona Antonia, did the cleaning. We were looking forward to moving in. Marilena also had another tenant called Biatriz. They were both very intelligent, well-travelled, cultured women. Bia was 29 and Marilena 49. She had two grown-up sons, one living in the USA and the other in São Paulo.

As Marilena showed us around the house with its cool white walls and terracotta tiled floor, she told us an old toad lived in the garden, but it was good for keeping down the bugs. Rebecca grinned at me. We stood on the verandah as the sun set and bats flew around the garden. Rebecca whispered, 'Mum, *look*!' and pointed to the bottom of the street where a monkey was clinging to a street lamp. 'This is *such* a cool place,' she breathed. I agreed. It was indeed. The garden was filled with the sound of cicadas instead of the noise of screeching buses and demolition crews that we heard from our apartment. We definitely wanted to live there.

Marilena invited us all to go to the cinema with her. We had to queue to buy tickets then we had to join another queue for 45 minutes to get into the theatre. The queue extended widthways as people strolled up to join their friends further up the line.

'This happens all the time here!' Marilena fumed.

Rebecca said, 'Oh, sod this,' and walked to the front of the queue. No one challenged her, but our English queuing protocol was too deeply ingrained for us to join her. When the doors opened there was a stampede. There were of course no seats left and I was not about to sit on the floor as many of the other luckless patrons were doing. Then we saw Rebecca waving from a row of empty seats she'd secured for us in the middle of the cinema.

'Well done,' Marilena congratulated her. 'You're becoming a Brazilian girl!'

Rebecca smiled proudly.

Next morning, back in New Zealand girl mode, she bought a saddle and bridle for her horse and a lead rope for the colt and we went off to the farm. Lilia and I lay in hammocks in front of the house, overlooking the lake, while Chris and David walked around the farm. Rebecca groomed her horses, stopping to laugh uproariously at the sight of a little puppy transporting itself around by clinging to the lower lip of a boxer. The parrot, Rosa, saw us and screeched from a nearby tree. Waltersede, the farm manager, had found him in his nest after his mother had been killed by dogs, Lilia said. Waltersede had taken him home and fed him every hour on porridge. Occasionally Rosa would yell, '*Ajuda!*' (Help!) in Waltersede's voice, causing everyone to run around in a panic. Often we saw him perched on Waltersede's head like a tattered, green hat.

'And why Rosa?' I asked, trailing a lazy leg out of the hammock.

'We thought he was a girl at first,' Lilia said, 'and when we found he was a boy, well the name just sorta suited him.'

Rebecca, Betsy and the two farm children went off to play volleyball, but Waltersede's goat wanted to join in. They tied him to a tree but the stench from the goat was enough to corrode the skin from our tonsils, so we left the hammocks and walked up to the house to sing happy birthday to the farm manager's boy, Valtier, and eat some birthday cake. Waltersede brought the goat too. He got lonely on his own, he explained. The goat smell was so overwhelmingly bad I had to go for a walk before I fainted from the fumes. Betsy and Rebecca made exaggerated gagging sounds, but Waltersede feigned incomprehension.

'What smell?' he shrugged.

A few weeks later, Waltersede found his way into a character study Rebecca wrote for an English assignment. She called it *Macho Man* and received an A for it. When I read this essay six years after she died, I wept for the hammocks, the goat and Rosa, and the casual assumptions of two 16-year-old girls playing volleyball by a bright blue lake under the hot Brazilian sun.

Marilia's sister, Magna, invited us to her wedding in Araguarí. Renato, a local boy Rebecca had turned down, was at the wedding. I saw him tense up when he saw Rebecca. He shook her hand and said hello stiffly. I felt sorry for him. Rebecca had lost interest in all the local boys now that she had a new love – her horse and colt. She preferred to spend her weekends picking ticks out of their ears with tweezers.

At Valerio's farm Leonardo and Evalbe caught and killed a metre-long poisonous snake and brought it to show us. Rebecca said it was beautiful. She stayed with the boys watching them put tags in the cows' ears while the rest of us went to the waterfall. After emerging from the warm water we lay on towels on the rocks gazing up at enormous spiders in webs that were strung out between the branches of trees. They were about a hand span in size and I wondered if they were waiting to catch flies or vultures.

At the end of this visit Rebecca wrote home:

Dear Momma, Susannah and Benjamin,

I've changed Troco's name to Beija-Flor. I didn't really like the name Troco. Also Cristiane is now called Cristy for short. On Saturday we bought a saddle, bridle and some other stuff for Cristy and a halter for Baby (the colt). The saddler is nothing like MacKenzies, the saddle and bridle is nothing like NZ saddlery but I'm getting used to the Brazilian style.

How are Song and Sing??? I hope they are as well as ever. Give them lots of cuddles and tell them I'll see them in just seven months' time.

Baby is so sweet. The name Beija-Flor is the Brazilian name for humming bird. It means Kiss-Flower and Baby has such a sweet face I decided to name him after a humming bird. Cristy is getting calmer every time I ride her. The farm is beautiful.

I really miss not having my cats with me. When I get back home I am going
to spend all my time with them!!!!!!!!!!!!!!!!!!!!!!!!!!

Well, got to go now, take care of my cats, say hi to everyone for me.

Tchau,

Your sis Beck

PS Don't believe Mum when she says I've lost interest in the local boys. I still
like Leonardo and when I went to a disco with Betsy there was a real cute guy
there dancing on one of the four stages around the room, with other guys. She
is right when she said I picked ticks out of the horses' ears. They were so gross.
They are green with horrible little legs sticking out everywhere. I had to squash
them with tweezers and blood and pus spattered out. I was nearly sick.

Several days later Rebecca and I were standing outside our apartment building at
6.30am. Reuben, who used to be a receptionist in our building, had invited us to visit the
school where he now taught English. He arrived half an hour late to pick us up. When
I got into the car the back of the seat fell off. There were no seatbelts, so I had to travel
sitting bolt upright. From the corner of my eye I could see Rebecca's shoulders quivering.
Reuben assured me he'd fix the seat with a bit of wood for the return journey. The dash-
board was held together with sticky tape and Reuben explained that was why he drove
very slowly, otherwise the car would fall apart.

At the traffic lights it started to roll backwards and whacked into a bus. Neither
Reuben nor the bus driver gave more than a passing glance at this occurrence. Reuben
told us it was his fourth car and the best he'd ever had. He liked it so much he'd brought
it from the Amazon on the back of a truck when he moved to Uberlândia last year. It
chugged along so slowly the other drivers on the road honked at us, but Reuben wasn't
worried. When we reached his school he said the secret of getting out of the car was to
wind down the window and open the door from the outside. Rebecca was bright red with
the effort of keeping her laughter in and I didn't dare look at her face or I would've lost
control myself.

We were welcomed to the school, which resembled a tin shed, by the principal and
deputy principal and taken to Reuben's class. Paint peeled off the dirty, bare walls of the
classrooms, which were crammed full of broken desks. The principal said they'd asked the
government for money for an upgrade, but had received only 25 per cent of what they'd
asked for. The teachers didn't get adequate salaries, she said, so they went on strike for

three or four months every year. Despite the appalling conditions, the students were happy and polite. They were bursting with questions about New Zealand and wanted to know if New Zealand boys had blond hair and blue eyes. The boys all wanted to know if Rebecca had a boyfriend. They crowded round her to get her autograph. She told them it was the first time she'd had rock star treatment. They asked us to come back again.

As we walked back to the car she asked Reuben in disbelief, 'Do they actually *like* that school?'

'Oh yes,' Reuben assured her. 'They feel lucky. Some children doesn't have a school to go to.'

After another hair-raising trip back to the apartment with the car falling apart around us, Rebecca and I maintained decorum long enough to walk sedately to the lift, but once inside we collapsed on the floor laughing. The lift stopped at the next floor and a man got in. We were mortified, but couldn't stop laughing. He got out hastily at the next floor. We staggered to our door and, safely inside, we threw ourselves on the bed, screaming with laughter.

'Oh *God*, Mum, your *face*, when the back of the seat fell off!' Rebecca shrieked.

As I looked at her doubled over, I was so glad she was here with us this year and that I had the opportunity to spend this time just with her. I wouldn't have missed this for the world, I thought.

'You'll tell this story to your kids one day,' I laughed.

The episode found its way into a short story I wrote called 'Bernardo's Car' and was broadcast on National Radio three years before Rebecca died. We listened to it together, Rebecca almost falling off her chair laughing at the memories it stirred. But that was four years in the future, when we still believed we had all the time in the world.

# THREE

# An owl lives here

On the night we moved into Marilena's house I went to do some washing and saw an enormous green creature, which I thought was a garden ornament. Then I remembered the giant toad Marilena had warned me about and sent Rebecca to see if it was breathing. She touched it and it blinked.

'It's *beautiful*, Mum!' she exclaimed, as I stood behind her, rejecting her invitation to examine it closely.

Chris was as fascinated as she was so I left them to it. When I told Marilena she assured me it couldn't jump. It was so fat it hardly moved at all, she said, and the gardener often had to shift it by moving it with his broom. When I told her I'd thought it was a garden ornament she laughed again because she'd never heard of toad garden ornaments and couldn't imagine why anyone would want such a thing.

The garden was regularly visited by parrots, toucans and thumb-sized humming birds. From the surrounding grasslands came the sounds of birds and cows, the occasional cackle of geese from the back garden, and Seu Pedro, who came in every day whistling as he trundled the wheelbarrow around the garden. Dona Antonia came twice a week to clean the windows and wash the floors.

The morning after we moved in I opened the shutters of our bedroom window and looked out at the garden. A branch from the mango tree extended right to our bedroom window. The dappled effects of the sun and shadow created a pattern along the length of the branch that looked like a supine woman with a stick through her heart. I called Chris to show him.

'Weird,' he said.

Later in the morning I walked around the garden and noticed the same dappled light and shadow effect in the trees. The patterns now seemed to resemble the faces of Brazilian Indians.

'Interesting trick of the light,' said Chris. 'Best not to say anything to Marilena. It might freak her out.'

Marilena saw me wandering around the garden and called me over to the mango tree. 'An owl lives here,' she said. 'Can you see?'

Just then the owl turned his head and looked at me.

'In Brazil some people believe they are symbols of death,' she said. 'Others believe they are lucky birds. Like guardians. So I'm very happy to have him live here in my tree.'

Chris's conference trip took us to São Paulo, Rio, the Amazon and Iguassu Falls. São Paulo: five million people, featureless buildings and no birds in the trees. Someone said it was because over-zealous spraying for insects had wiped out the food sources for the birds. A group of handsome young engineering students were assigned to guide us round the city. In the snake house Rebecca asked what snakes ate. 'Tender young teenage girls,' said one of the delegates. Everyone laughed as Rebecca rolled her eyes. The boys promised to take her to a spider house next. Our bus slammed on its brakes. Screeching wheels on slippery tarmac. A cacophony of cars honking. Drivers winding down windows, shouting. We strained to see through the smeared windows. A bundle of rags in a puddle of yellow light in the middle of the rain-slicked road. The bundle moved. It had a head and arms, but no legs. And it was shaking its fists. More shouting. More honking. Cars revved their engines, swerved around the bundle and went on their way. The legless man finally pulled himself over to the pavement, and sat there shaking his fists at the world. Rebecca's hands flew to her mouth. A woman in the opposite seat leaned over to touch her arm. 'Is a beggar,' she said, shaking her head. 'Happens a lot here.'

In São Paulo Rebecca turned 17.

Narrow mountain roads. Valleys covered with palms and banana trees. The driver overtaking trucks on hairpin bends only to arrive in Rio at rush hour. Determined to get us to our hotel in time he ricocheted off pavements, scattering pedestrians and hurtled the wrong way down one-way streets.

Rio: Copacabana with its impossibly beautiful people in impossibly minute swimwear on white, curved beaches. The beach at São Conrado. 'This one is safer,' said the guide. 'But don't wear any jewellery or watches.'

Sugar Loaf Mountain at sunset. The navy blue sky shot through with gold. The lights around the bays strung like jewels on a necklace. The café where Jobin wrote 'Girl from Ipanema'. Rebecca laughing, having her photograph superimposed beside one of Tom Cruise and printed on a T-shirt. Rebecca cruising the shopping malls with me, the museums and art galleries. The Rodin exhibition. Rebecca engrossed in scribbling notes about the exhibits for her Art History course.

'So d'you think it's better than last time you were here?'

'Yeah. But I still prefer the farm.'

And then the *favelas*. Hundreds of filthy shacks of corrugated iron and wood stacked precariously up the hillsides. 'Is where the most famous samba schools come from,' said the guide. 'They spend all the year preparing for the *Carnaval* in February. You must come back to Rio then to see it. Is one of the wonders of the world.'

Rebecca staring at the snotty-nosed children and mangy dogs in the rubbish-filled streets and falling silent. The guide noticing. 'Well, at least they get one of the best views in Rio,' he offered. When the bus stopped at a gem shop he told us to remain seated until the guards arrived and escorted us inside. 'Is just for the security.'

On the way to Corcovada to see the Christ statue our taxi driver crossed himself every time it came into view as he charged round corners. Was he religious or trying to protect himself from his own maniacal driving? The funicular ride through the hibiscus-filled Tijuca Forest with its enormous red and blue butterflies. The Christ statue at the top from where we looked down on Sugar Loaf.

'It's like standing on top of the world,' I said. 'Worth that taxi ride, d'you reckon?'

Rebecca nodded. 'Yeah. It's okay.'

The Amazon. The rainforest like a vast sea of broccoli. The Opera House in Manaus, its richly carved interior, imported marble, velvet and crystal a testimony to the wealth of the rubber boom. Its collapse was manifest in the city of Manaus, in its seething mass of people, blaring radios, screaming advertising vans, beggars waggling their stumps at passers-by, men hoiking and spitting in the streets, graffiti-splattered buildings and piles of putrid rubbish rotting in the hot, humid air.

The black water of the Rio Negro and the pale brown water of the Solimões mingled in a plaited pattern for 18 kilometres until they merged into the chocolate brown of the Amazon River. In the jungle, monkeys swung through the trees and scarlet parrots shrieked. A grey bird flew over our canoe with a long, thin snake dangling from its beak. Clusters of white birds frothed the tops of trees like apple blossom. Luminous blue butterflies flitted in the bars of pale green light that slanted through the dense overhang of trees and creepers. Giant water lilies floated on the water.

'This is *amazing*, Mum,' Rebecca whispered.

'Better than Rio?'

'Oh, *God* yes!'

In a clearing on the river bank a little girl showed us her pet sloth. A man standing beside a giant kapok tree brought over a python. We took a photograph of Rebecca wearing it over her shoulders and another of her holding a tiny monkey. At a stall in another clearing, Indian feathered necklaces, masks, and varnished piranha fish on sticks were on sale. They, along with the hundreds of butterflies encased in glass paperweights and displayed on plates and trays on the shelves of the tourist shops, found their way into Rebecca's Art History essay on the effects of tourism on indigenous crafts.

Iguassu Falls straddle the Brazilian and Argentinian borders. The jet boat took us to the bottom of the falls where multiple rainbows circled the cascading waters while we screamed with delight at riding the rapids and getting soaking wet. At the bottom of the valley little raccoon-like creatures called *coatis* clambered over the rocks and a thousand species of butterflies fluttered in the jungle.

At the conference dinner Rebecca won a bottle of Gucci perfume. When her name was called she blushed and was reluctant to walk up to the stage to collect it, but the applause from everyone else encouraged her to do so.

'There you go,' grinned Chris. 'Just like a *real* girl.'

Dear Susannah, Benjamin, Sing and Song,

   Hi, how are you? The holiday was excellent. I liked São Paulo the best. We went on a tour and three university boys showed us around the city. One, who offered to take me to the spider farm, was gorgeous. He looked just like Sylvester Stallone. I didn't like Rio much but it was okay. Manaus was pretty cool, especially the trip through the Amazon. I loved holding the snake. It was very heavy and it felt like that big plastic lizard Benjamin had. It wasn't slimy like people think. There were lots of big brightly coloured birds for you Sing, and heaps of piranha for you to fish Song.

Thank you for the birthday card and email. Unfortunately the card was very chewed and soggy.

Well that's all from me, Take care of my cats.

Tchau,

Rebecca

I sat on the verandah watching the light deepen and fill the garden with purple shadows. A flock of green and red parrots flew screeching past and a toucan landed heavily on a branch. It looked like a glove puppet with a varnished yellow beak.

Rebecca called from her hammock, 'Mum! Look!' and pointed to a bumble bee-sized humming-bird whirring around the orchids.

'*Beija-Flor*,' said Seu Pedro, and got her to repeat the pronunciation after him. She did so, the picture of indolence in her hammock, not telling him she already knew.

'Seu Pedro,' I said in my halting Portuguese, 'you won't believe this, but she's working very hard in there.'

'I am! I am!' Rebecca grinned.

Seu Pedro doubled over laughing. It felt nice, sharing a joke in Portuguese.

Marilena told us her ex-husband had been a political prisoner in Brazil in the early 1970s, during the time of the military government. She said at that time the military police arrested thousands of people, especially students and lecturers. They just appeared in the classrooms and took people away. Some were never seen again. Thousands of young people were killed. When her husband got out of prison they went to the USA for three years, where they worked on a political magazine to let people know what was happening in Latin America, which was almost all under military government at that time. Their visa ran out after three years, but they couldn't go back to Brazil or her husband would have been arrested. Instead, they went to Chile. After a year, there was a military coup and thousands of Brazilians who had escaped to Chile were arrested. She described the terror of seeing tanks roll up to people's houses and take them away. 'They became "the disappeared". No one dared talk about them,' she said. She and her husband escaped and when they went back to Brazil he went into hiding till an amnesty was declared for political prisoners.

The house she lived in had been designed by her husband and herself based on the best places they'd ever lived in. It was eco-friendly and had been the realisation of a long-held dream. Her husband had a job at the university and she began her PhD. However, their marriage foundered and they divorced. Her 16-year-old son, Marcelo, had gone to complete his education in the USA, where he'd been born. Bruno, born in Brazil, would have gone too, she said, if he'd been lucky enough to have US citizenship. Now, as well as being Head of Department and finally completing her disrupted PhD, she was an active environmentalist and part of a team surveying and recording the flora and fauna of a valley that would soon be flooded. She went off on field trips into the wilds and brought back orchids, which she cultivated in her garden, and sometimes rocks and crystals. I liked her immensely.

Bia worked for the telephone company and spent her time between Uberlândia and São Paulo, so she was not in the house very often. She lived with an artist in São Paulo when she was there, but he'd just gone off on an extended trip to Europe to exhibit his paintings.

Bruno had now finished his degree in computer science and would be staying at home till the end of the year. He wanted to begin his MSc the following year. The house was big enough to accommodate us all very comfortably.

In June the whole of Brazil was busy celebrating the festivals of São Antonio and São João with bonfires, fireworks and street parties. Marilia invited Bruno and us to a farm in Goiás, a tiny town about 100 kilometres away, for the San João festival. The farm, belonging to Marilia's relatives, was set in a plantation of banana and mango trees, corn and sugar cane. It was 90 years old and was a rabbit warren of dark rooms with tiny windows that let in almost no light.

All the relatives and friends had been invited, including the one policeman and ambulance driver from the nearest town with a population of 600. We all crowded into a small yard under a roof of bamboo leaves to keep out of the blazing midwinter sun. Enormous cauldrons of rice, beans, manioc, pork, chicken and beef steamed on wooden tables.

As we began to eat, a brass band came into the middle of the yard and started playing. I thought I'd adapted to the noise level in Brazil, but this was a cacophony on a scale hitherto unimagined. The effect was like being inside a concrete mixer full of fire sirens. My brain experienced meltdown in about 30 seconds and Chris and I had to get up and move ourselves to a safer distance, though Rebecca didn't appear to notice the noise. After the meal, pictures of the saints were hoisted on long poles decorated with streamers and oranges, firecrackers were set off and bonfires lit. The heat was akin to landing on the sun.

That night we went to a São João party at the Country Club in Araguarí. At the party bright streamers, paper lanterns and bamboo decorated the walls and ceiling. A band played country-and-western music and people danced, ate corn and manioc and drank hot mulled wine. Bruno, Rebecca and Evalbe met up with more of their friends and danced all evening. Finally at 1.30am we left, though people were still arriving. The party would go on all night.

On the way home Rebecca said, 'I'm so glad we came to Brazil.'

'So am I,' I said. 'In future years, you'll always have friends to visit here. People who will welcome you and keep you safe.'

# FOUR

# A ring of burning candles

Despite Rebecca's protestations that Correspondence School was 'the pits', the graph of grades for her work she'd pinned above her desk continued to rise. In English she had to build up a folio of her own writing. Many of her essays sprang from her feelings of alienation and then acceptance as a foreigner in a culture very different to her own. To her surprise the teacher asked for two of her short stories and an essay to go in the Correspondence School magazine.

As a child she had drawn horses and other animals and had written captions to illustrate the pictures. As she got older the captions lengthened into stories. The stories usually had the same theme of a young animal losing its mother or becoming separated from the herd, but somehow managing to save the world. As I worked at the computer on my own writing, Rebecca would sprawl on the floor of my study working on hers. From time to time we would read each other excerpts of our work. The writing she showed me in Brazil surprised me with its depth and humour. After we got back to New Zealand, however, she let the writing drop and focused her energy on her drawing and painting. I continued reading my own stories to her before I wrote the final drafts. She was the only person I ever read them to and she was frank in her criticism: 'What on earth was *that* about?' and generous with her praise: 'Hey, that's *cool*, Mum!'

Chris and Rebecca came back from the farm and brought with them a clump of matted black hair from a horse's tail. Rebecca put it behind the chair where I'd been working and called me out to look at it. She said it was a giant caterpillar. I leapt out of my chair and they fell about laughing. Then she played the same joke on Marilena. She put it near the CD player and asked Marilena what it was.

'I've no idea!' gasped Marilena. 'Wait! I'll get a torch. In the meantime, open the door so it can get out.'

Rebecca's delighted shrieks alerted her to the joke and she joined in the laughter, flushed with relief.

Bruno took Rebecca to a graduation party. She had no dress to wear so went in her jeans. Next day it was Marilena's birthday. We spent all day cooking and preparing for the party. We lit candles and put them around the garden and house. The party began at 9pm and finished at 3am. Even Rebecca was feeling a bit jaded by then, but we enjoyed sitting on the verandah in the warm evening air, being encouraged in our attempts to speak Portuguese by Marilena's guests. Rebecca admired Bia's beautiful black designer dress and Bia immediately said she could borrow it for the next graduation party. Rebecca tried it on and looked gorgeous in it, but declined Bia's offer. The step from jeans to dresses was too big to take just yet.

Bruno bought a new white Chevrolet and invited suggestions for its name. Rebecca came up with Brunomobile so that became its name for the decade that he kept it. He now had to sell his motorbike. Before doing this he asked Rebecca if she would like a ride. My fretting about the dangers of motorbikes only convinced her to ride it, but I warned Bruno not to go too fast. He took Rebecca over the hills around the neighbourhood and later told me she'd kept telling him to go faster, but he hadn't dared because of my warning. 'If something happened to her I knew you would never forgive me,' he said, and I loved him for it.

Bruno was beautiful with big brown eyes and black curly hair. He was also uncharacteristically shy for a Brazilian, so I tried to draw him out by besieging him with questions about Brazil. He answered me very patiently and gradually got used to having us living in the house. He seemed to eat nothing but pizza and popcorn. The day he cooked up a batch of popcorn and invited us to share it with him in the kitchen was the day I knew he'd accepted us. From then on the popcorn cook-ups became a regular occurrence. If Bia was home she would join us and send Bruno and Rebecca into paroxysms of laughter with tales of her travels.

Rebecca asked Bruno to help her find out how *pamonha* was made for a school project. He took her around all the places he knew in Uberlândia, but nobody would divulge the secret. When Dona Antonia got to hear of this she threw up her hands. 'Why didn't you ask *me?*' After that she sat at the table and explained the whole process with Bruno translating and Rebecca writing it all down. When the results were returned a few weeks later with an A for the project, I told Dona Antonia it was she who had got the A. She laughed and laughed.

Bruno also took Rebecca to art supplies shops to find whatever she needed for various art projects. His patience with her requests was endless. They started going to the movies together. Bia opined that Bruno was falling in love with Rebecca.

'Poor Bruno,' said Chris. 'He'll have to grow a mane and a tail.'

Marilena arranged a weekend in Caldas Novas, a hot springs area in Goiás, for us all. The scenery was typical *Cerrado* – very dry with twisted black *sucupira* trees and *burriti* palms. We arrived as the sun went down and the sky blazed blood red.

In the evening we swam under a full moon. I observed how Bruno looked at Rebecca and concluded that Bia was right. Rebecca, however, was oblivious.

Dear Benjamin,

Hi, how are you and Dee? I'm okay and so are Cristy and Beija-Flor, my two horses. Cristy is going to have another foal but I'll never see it because I'll be back in New Zealand. How are Sing and Song? I'm glad to hear that Song is better now, why was she sick before? Have you seen any bald patches on her?

Everyone here in Brazil thinks I'm strange because I ride and muck about with horses. All the girls here are so weak and feeble and the guys are macho and think that horses are a man's job. It's great fun watching their reaction when I can handle horses better than them.

All the men think that a horse has to be bashed about and abused and when I bought Cristy she would always run away from people because she thought that she was going to be hit, but now she waits for me. Beija-Flor (humming bird) always comes up to me and rests his head in my arms. He is so cute. He is one and a half. He's Cristy's son. Cristy is 16 years old.

So what's been happening in NZ? What's the weather like? Amber has told me it was snowing. Here it is winter and is only 30 degrees. (How cold). It's the dry season and all the grass is going brown so the horses are getting thin (not my horses because they get fed but David's 38 horses).

Has Mum told you about the fires that people light every winter? The countryside is dotted with burnt grass and fires. The smell of smoke is everywhere. For some reason the people who light the fires think that if they don't set the grass on fire it won't grow again next summer.

We've just got back from a trip to Caldas Novas, hot springs. The water is really hot. And so is the sun, so it is impossible to escape the heat.

Well, that's all I can think of to say, take care of my cats, say hi to everyone for me.

Tchau,

Beck

PS I wish you were here.

At a conference in Uberlândia on Afro-Brazilian religious cults, the city council was negotiating with the leaders of the cults to get their members to clean up after they'd performed their rituals at waterfalls and rivers. They used those places for *Macumba* ceremonies and the riverbanks got littered with offerings of food, black candles and sacrificed animals, which was off-putting for tourists, the council argued.

The crossroads and waterfalls near Marilena's house were also used for *Macumba* ceremonies. One night we heard drums beating and next morning, as we were driving into town, we saw a black chicken, a bowl of rice and a bottle of wine lying in the middle of the crossroads.

'*Macumba*,' said Marilena.

I jumped out of the car to take a photograph.

'No! Don't touch it!' she called.

I asked if she was superstitious.

'Of course not, but somebody might be watching,' she claimed, not very convincingly.

*Macumba* had arrived with the slaves from Africa and involved both black and white magic. When I started asking Marilena questions about it she said she would try to find someone who could take me to a ceremony. For several weeks I'd been going to Marilena's masseuse, Marlí, because of problems with my neck. Marlí would know more about *Macumba* than she did, said Marilena. That turned out to be true and the stories she told me helped my Portuguese progress more quickly than my grammar book and weekly lessons.

Bruno and Rebecca said they'd seen a ring of burning candles on the road one night as they were driving to the cinema. Rebecca, however, was more interested in the film,

*Braveheart*, and loved it so much they went back to see it the next night. She played the soundtrack of the film constantly.

Seven years later we would play it at her funeral.

On the verandah we drank wine and beer and ate *pão de queixo* that Marilena baked. Bia played the guitar and she and Marilena sang. One song was 'London, London', which Caetano Velosa had written during his three-year exile in London after the military coup in Brazil.

Marilena said, 'No one likes to talk of it now. But that was a dark period of our history.'

We sat in silence for a while as dusk fell. Then Bia said, 'Sandra, Chris, Rebecca, in a few months you will be gone from here. Do you think you can leave us, just like that?'

To my surprise I couldn't answer her through the sudden rush of tears.

Marilena said, 'But you *will* come back, won't you? Bia and I will always be here. This house will always be a home for you.'

'Yes, we'll be back,' I answered, sad at how quickly the year was slipping away. Soon all this would be just a memory. What would have happened in our lives by the next time we sat here, I wondered.

Dear Susannah and Mark,

Hi, how RU? I'm great. Tomorrow I'm going to see *Lancelot, First Knight* for the third time. It is the BEST movie ever!! I didn't think *Braveheart* was very gruesome. It was an excellent movie too. How's your new flat? Have you been round to our house and checked that Sing and Song are being looked after properly?

I can't wait until it rains here because it is so hot and dry and all the grass is dead and the horses are getting so thin. I miss the frosty mornings and snow and hail and rain of NZ, believe it or not.

Have you seen pictures of Cristy and Beija-Flor? Well I've put some in this letter. They are pretty thin and scrawny looking but that's because there's no feed for them.

Well, got to go now. See you soon (in just 85 days)

Tchau

Rebecca

# FIVE

# Leaving Brazil

Ouro Preto is a historic city in Minas Gerais, named after the gold that was discovered there in the 18th century. The Jesuit priests insisted it be used to build extravagant churches. The city belongs to UNESCO and nothing can be altered. It is, therefore, a time capsule of Baroque architecture. We were visiting it so that Rebecca could write about it for her Art History project. The city is in the mountains, so the streets are narrow and steep and cobblestoned, with little houses and inns on either side, like an illustration from *Grimm's Fairy Tales*. At night, the valley is dotted with lights and the sound of church bells floats in the air.

Chris and I were enchanted with the city, the religious art museum and the churches. By the third day, however, Rebecca had seen enough of gold angels and suffering saints to last her a lifetime.

'Not more bloody churches!' she said as we suggested one final visit.

'Think of your Art History project,' I reminded her.

She groaned.

She was desperate for civilisation. When we returned to Belo Horizonte, the capital of the state, we let her cruise the highly sophisticated shopping malls. But the only thing she bought was a red halter for her horse.

We'd arranged to meet Fabiano, the young medical student/waiter we'd met in Porto Seguro in February. He showed us around Belo Horizonte and invited us to his uncle's barbecue in the evening. His relatives greeted us like old friends, and I enjoyed watching the way the family members all hugged and kissed each other. Fabiano picked up his two-year-old cousin and hugged him tight. How loved the children in this society must feel, I thought. He told us he was in two choirs and that music and medicine were like two halves of his soul. He felt complete when he could do both. Though he'd just turned 22 he seemed older than his years and we were very impressed with him. As we said goodbye, he said he'd like to come and visit us in Uberlândia the following week.

Rebecca had two more weeks to go before she finished her Correspondence School course. After that, she wanted to spend her remaining weeks studying Portuguese. Terezinha arranged lessons three times a week for her with three other foreign students. She also wanted to go to the farm two days during the week as well as weekends, so she could train more horses.

Dona Antonia invited us for lunch and asked Bruno to go with us to translate. Her husband had bought a fish in the market that morning and she'd gone to a lot of trouble to prepare the meal and arrange it artistically. Her husband brought out a dish of water and a pink soap with the wrapping still on so we could wash our hands. Marilena later told us this was so we would realise the soap was new. Normally they did not buy soap as Dona Antonia made her own.

After the meal she took us up the street to meet her mother who lived in an even worse shack with just one room that contained a bed, a chair and a stove. Dozens of children, ducklings and goats ran in and out of the house where Dona Antonia's mother greeted us all very warmly, and her daughters piled around her bed, some with babies. Rebecca, to her credit, took a turn at holding one of the babies and making admiring noises.

Dona Antonia gave me a bar of the soap she'd been making the last time I visited her. She held up the soap to the light and said, 'When you saw me making this it was so brown and ugly, Dona Sandra. But see now how beautiful it is.'

I told her I'd love to put her in my suitcase and take her back to New Zealand. She said she'd love to come. I did put her in a short story several years later.

Rebecca asked Seu Pedro if he knew where she could dig up a few worms. She tried to explain to him in Portuguese that she needed some for her biology project. She'd tried a few places in the garden, but couldn't find any. Seu Pedro mentioned this to his son, who went to the riverbed and returned with a bucket full of worms. He presented this to Rebecca with great pride and was very disappointed when we explained she needed only a few.

Rebecca took a worm to the kitchen and began to read what she had to do with it. A shriek of indignation. 'What! No *way*! It says here, before dissecting your worm, *boil* it!'

After all the trouble Seu Pedro's son had gone to, the report she wrote for her worm project was mostly fiction. Soon after that, Seu Pedro's son had to escape into the *favelas* in Rio to avoid a court case in which he was charged with fatally shooting a neighbour. When Bruno visited us in New Zealand three years later he said the boy returned for a family visit and was shot dead by avenging relatives. But all that was still in the future.

Fabiano arrived by overnight bus from Belo Horizonte. The next day we went to the farm to join David, Lilia and Betsy, a couple of Betsy's friends, and a couple of David's agricultural students for a barbecue. Rebecca saddled up the horses for herself, Bruno and Fabiano to ride. Fabiano offered to help, but she brusquely elbowed him out of the way. He opened the gate for her and she scowled, 'I'm not helpless!' Fabiano raised startled eyebrows. Bruno smiled to himself.

The rainy season was just starting and in the afternoon the rain fell in solid sheets. Rebecca jumped into the lake in her shorts calling out that she loved the rain. The rest of us ran into the farmhouse. Two hours later we were still there talking, laughing and singing English and Portuguese songs.

When we got back home, Marilena brought out freshly baked *pão de caixo* for us and we all sat in the kitchen eating, drinking and listening to music. So much laughter. So much conversation. I told Marilena I loved the way Brazilians laughed so much.

She said, 'But Sandra, I've never heard anyone laugh as much as you, Chris and Rebecca. I've never seen a family as happy as you three.'

I reflected that Brazil had given us the time and space out of our busy lives not just to be happy, but just to *be*, and for that I would always be grateful.

The following evening we took Fabiano and Bruno to an outdoor café for a pizza and then to an ice-cream shop. Rebecca was telling the boys how feeble she thought Brazilian girls were. 'Why, they can't even open a farm gate!'

Fabiano asked her, with a slight edge to his voice, how come New Zealand girls were so tough.

'We have a strong feminist movement in New Zealand,' she said.

Bruno burst out laughing. 'A few weeks ago you said feminists were all lesbians with hairy legs!'

'Well, okay, I exaggerated!' she retorted.

They said if she was so tough she should go and stand in the rain as she obviously liked rain so much. At that moment a group of girls in high heels and miniskirts huddled in the doorway to shelter from the downpour. When it eased a few minutes later, a man opened the door for them and they teetered out, giggling.

Rebecca burst out laughing. 'See what I mean! *Pathetic!*'

Bruno laughed. Fabiano frowned and told her she shouldn't generalise about Brazilian girls. She shrugged.

On Sunday we took Fabiano to the bus station for his nine-hour return journey to Belo Horizonte. It felt like saying goodbye to an old and dear friend. He said he'd come to visit us in New Zealand one day.

'Mum, he had tears in his eyes,' Rebecca said in disbelief. 'Brazilians are so … so … *I* don't know!'

Over the next seven years she would see his tears many times.

A couple of days later Bia came back from her six-week trip to the USA. She brought her boyfriend, Luiz. The visit was well timed because Rebecca was able to interview him for an art project. He brought some photographs of his paintings to show her and when she chose one she liked he took it into the city to get a colour photocopy of it and signed it for her. His paintings were impressionist and delicate. Luiz was very interesting and funny, so we had another good few days of eating, drinking and talking till the early hours.

We posted off the final package for Rebecca's Correspondence School course. When the results of her exams came back she was amazed to find how well she'd done and forgot to be cool as she waved the piece of paper at me, even enduring my delighted hugs and kisses.

While Luiz was still with us we all decided to spend a morning by a beautiful river about 20 kilometres out of the city. Despite the *Macumba* offerings on the bank, the place felt very peaceful with its waterfall, birdsong and cicadas. Chris went for a walk and the others went exploring while I stayed in the water, swimming. When they came back they got into the water with me. Chris said he'd returned earlier than he intended because he'd felt very uncomfortable in the area, as if he were being watched. He didn't like the place at all. He said he thought he'd heard voices around him and rationalised it must have been the sound of the river. Luiz said he'd discovered a cave behind the waterfall in which he'd sensed the lives of many generations of people who'd lived there thousands of years before. Marilena said she'd felt she was invading the privacy of the spirits of nature, so mentally she'd asked permission to be there and felt at ease. I felt none of this and simply enjoyed the peace and beauty of the place.

Later in the day, while we were having lunch in the city, Luiz talked about the manifestations of spirits of nature. Marilena talked about the spirits around her home that many people had sensed. Because of this I felt able to tell her that when we'd first moved into her house I'd seen shadow and light dappling the trees in the garden and had been struck at how the patterns they formed resembled the faces of Indians. Marilena said that Indians had in fact lived around that area centuries earlier and what I'd seen might have been guardians of the land.

Rebecca looked at me and rolled her eyes.

Dear Susannah and Benjamin,

Well I for one will definitely not be sorry to leave Brazil. I can't wait to get back to NZ!! Although I'll miss the farm. Finally I've finished Correspondence School. Yehah!!! But now I have to learn Portuguese three times a week! (by myself!!) how boring!!!

Mum has completely cracked this year. She's seeing Indians in the trees and believes in spirits!

In your last letter you gave amazing advice – try buying food for your horses. Of course I buy food for them but the man who is supposed to be feeding them may or may not feed them. David reckons he gives the horse food to his cows.

But anyway, HAPPY BIRTHDAY!!! Hope you had a great birthday. What did you do?

Well, got to go. Have fun.

Rebecca

PS You'll look great in a bikini.

Rebecca had worked miracles with her horse. Now it trotted up to her whinnying softly – usually accompanied by the gander whose wife had been eaten by something in the lake. The poor creature was obviously lonely because it never left the horse's side. Whenever we saw Rebecca riding the horse, accompanied by the foal and a line of other horses, we expected to see the gander bringing up the rear.

David said he'd buy Beija-Flor for the riding school and someone was interested in buying Cristiane. Rebecca couldn't bear the thought of leaving them behind and had been trying hard to persuade Chris to bring the two horses to New Zealand, but we convinced her that with quarantine regulations, not to mention the expense, it would be impractical. David said he'd keep her busy with training the other horses. The building for the riding school was about to start; the trainers were working with the horses and new foals were being born. It was a wonderful opportunity for Rebecca to see it all grow and know she had a small part to play in its development. She sometimes had races with the vets and David's agronomy students and, invariably winning, she enjoyed the reputation she developed for her daring.

On the opposite bank of the lake to the farmhouse there was some mud which was the kind offered in expensive beauty salons. One day I lay in the sun with the mud smeared all over my skin watching Rebecca chasing Bruno with handfuls of the oozy stuff. Fastidious boy that he was, he didn't let her catch him. I could hear his protests and Rebecca's shrieks of laughter. Scissor-tails scooted over the surface of the lake catching insects. The horses wandered down for a drink. Waltersede ambled over to his house with Rosa perched on his head, screeching. '*Ajuda!*' I could see Chris and David working on the new track. The sun blazed out of a brilliant blue sky. I closed my eyes. *Hold this moment. Hold it. Hold it. Hold it. Hold it. Hold it.*

Rebecca stayed for two nights at the farm with Betsy and her friend. The sheeting rain didn't stop the girls going out on a three-hour trek. They all slept together in one room as they were the only ones on the farm and it was very isolated. I worried about snakes, vampire bats and tarantula spiders, but Rebecca thought it a great adventure.

'Mum, I saw this *enormous*, hairy spider in the water trough. It was so *beautiful.*'

'Spider and beautiful is an oxymoron!'

'And a bright green frog with red eyes in the bathroom. So *cool!*'

'Omigod!'

And I watched her as she ran off to the lake, tanned legs leaping over the grass, blonde hair flying behind her, as amazed by her as I had been ever since she was a child.

In the laundry at Marilena's house Bruno suddenly yelled out, 'Rebecca, be careful!' and pointed to a scorpion only centimetres from her bare foot.

'Oops!' she laughed and bent close to inspect it. Seu Pedro took it away and brought a dead one from the shed to show us. He'd pickled it in alcohol and said this was the best antidote for scorpion bites. He also brought in a large green and turquoise lizard, which one of the dogs had chewed, to show Rebecca and promised to look out for a snake for her. I told Dona Antonia we didn't have snakes in New Zealand. She greeted this news with disbelief. 'No snakes? You must live in paradise.'

We'd arrived in Uberlândia in the rainy season when the Christmas lights decorated the city. Now once more the rainy season had begun and the *Cerrado* was turning from black after the burn-offs to bright green. The flame trees glowed again with huge, crimson flowers. Lights were going up in the city and they'd be switched on a couple of days before we left. Everything was completing its cycle. Even the giant toad came wobbling across the garden.

'It's come to say goodbye to you, Mum!' Rebecca laughed.

The farewell parties began. At our last barbecue on Valerio's farm, Leonardo and Evalbe came with us to the waterfall. Rebecca decided she wasn't going to swim so the boys grabbed her and threw her in the river. They showed her how to use the rocks as a slide. Sebastião captured this on video.

'She's changed a lot since she first came here,' Marilia observed as we watched them all shrieking with laughter.

Dear S and M,

Mum is calling my horse an 'it' but she is a SHE! Sometimes I have races with the guys at the farm (I ride Skewbald, a beautiful Skewbald brown and white mare). She is so fast and I can beat everyone in races. João (the horse trainer) challenged me to a race and he was riding Jurubeba, a grey mare and I was on Skewbald and he whipped his horse and yelled like a cowboy trying to beat me and Skewy, but ha ha we won!! João had to swallow his machismo and even managed to say 'Congratulations!' Me and Skewy are unbeatable!

When I went to Araguari we went to a swimming hole in a river. I didn't want to go swimming because I didn't want to get changed. Leonardo and Evalbe decided that I would go swimming and threw me in the water (in my jeans!). Fortunately they took off my watch and shoes (Gee, how kind of them!) So in the end I had to get changed anyway.

Oh yeah, Mum's called Beija-Flor a foal but he's a two year old!

Anyway better go.

See ya soon.

Tchau,

Rebecca

The last barbecue at David's farm. We took a photo of Bruno and Rebecca standing on the branch of a tree that hung low over the cracked red earth. We sat in the car and waited while Rebecca said goodbye to Cristiane and Beija-Flor. Her head was bent over the horse's mane and I knew she was crying.

David, Lilia and Betsy, Marilena and Bruno, Sebastião and Marilia and Camacho came to the airport to say goodbye. To our amazement, Calvino turned up too and gave us a video of one of his concert performances. He stayed till it was time for us to get on the plane. Marilena hugged us and turned away to leave. It was very hard to watch her go.

Sebastião gave us the video he'd been taking of our year in Brazil. 'So you will always remember us.'

We said goodbye to these dear people who'd been so kind and hospitable. The only one who didn't have wet eyes was Rebecca.

The plane rose higher over Uberlândia. When would we be back? Not too long, I hoped.

Rebecca leaned forward in her seat. 'I promised David I'd go back and help him with his riding school. Maybe when I've finished seventh form.' And she settled back and began to talk about the horse she'd buy as soon as we got home. She asked if we could move from Christchurch to the country. She'd like to be able to see her horse from her bedroom window. Just like on David's farm.

# SIX

# Back to New Zealand

Back in New Zealand, Rebecca's first priority was to look for another horse. Within a week we bought Lace, a grey mare, and installed her in a paddock close to home. After the summer Rebecca went back to Burnside High School for her seventh form year. Most of the students she'd associated with before leaving for Brazil had already left school and she was dismayed at the prospect of making new friends all over again. However, with her tanned skin, sun-streaked blonde hair and the new confidence she'd gained in Brazil, she discovered that she was, once again, the centre of attention and interest.

Two names that cropped up a lot in Rebecca's conversations over the next few months were Bart and Grant. I met them when she threw her first party. They were both tall, lanky boys with a great sense of humour, judging by the gales of laughter I heard from Rebecca every time she talked to them on the phone. Natasha, one of her closest friends, had already left school, but they'd kept in contact during the year and now Natasha joined the ever-growing crowds of young people who trooped through our house. Although she'd never ridden before, Natasha decided to start riding lessons, and she and Rebecca scoured the ads looking for a suitable horse. They eventually found a 15-year-old chestnut gelding thoroughbred, which they named Red, and moved him to a paddock next to Lace.

After a few weeks Rebecca said, 'I never thought I'd ever say this but I love school, I love the subjects I'm studying, and I love all my teachers.'

I looked at her with an eyebrow raised.

'Well, all the teachers except the old bag!'

There were many changes in the air. Susannah had moved into a flat while we were in Brazil and when we returned home I couldn't get used to the sight of her empty room. Within a few days Benjamin got engaged to his girlfriend, Dee, on her 21st birthday and moved into a flat with her.

Years before, I had lain in bed one morning, listening to the music, laughter and chatter of my children and estimated how many more years I'd still have them before the house emptied. Now the emptying had begun. Friends assured me the empty nest was a great stage of life, once you got used to it. Although Susannah and Benjamin dropped by frequently, Rebecca missed having them in the house. 'I don't want to be an only one,' she complained. 'You'll both gang up on me now.'

Apart from the quietness and empty spaces in our big old house, every time I left it I was struck by the quietness, emptiness and cleanliness of the streets. I longed for the noise, the heat, the music and the exuberance of Brazilian streets, the smiles, the greetings and the warmth of the people. Chris felt the same, but Rebecca had no such sentimental attachment.

'I sure don't miss the pong of dead animals,' she said, though conceded that she did miss David's farm.

Over the following year my *saudades* for Brazil were slowly absorbed into the process of getting established in my new job, enjoying the company of our friends again and organising Susannah's wedding.

Susannah and Mark got married at the end of 1996 and Benjamin and Dee at the beginning of 1997. Rebecca started Lincoln University soon after to study Farm Management, got her driver's licence and bought a car. After suffering several strokes Chris's mother needed 24-hour care and she decided it was time to go into a resthome. Where originally there'd been seven of us, Chris, Rebecca and I were now rattling around in our big, empty, old house, which would soon be due for some serious maintenance. We were dismayed to see that some of the beautiful old villas in our street had been demolished, and ugly town houses were springing up in their place. Since living in Brazil, Rebecca had been keen to move to the country so she could keep her horse in a paddock within sight of her bedroom window. We weighed up the inconvenience of commuting for an hour to work each day with the assault on our sanity of yet more noisy neighbours. A nearby party with bagpipes wailing in the garden at 3am and all-night parties in the houses on either side of us convinced us commuting was the healthier option.

We found a beautiful cottage in North Canterbury within an hour's commute to town and moved in at the end of April. A few days later, Lace and Red arrived and Rebecca at last achieved her dream of having her horse close by.

We couldn't believe we owned this beautiful house overlooking farmland, with the snowy peaks of the Southern Alps as our backdrop, and spent the first few weeks feeling as if we were on holiday. Rebecca spent most of her time in the old barn arranging a tack room and putting up horse pictures to decorate it. She called me in to look at her handiwork. She was wearing a pair of shorts and a bikini top and as we went into the paddock to catch her horse she started skipping, her two Siamese cats running behind her, erect tails waving like flags in the long grass.

I smiled at her. 'You're happy, aren't you?'

She grinned and hugged herself.

She had just turned 19.

I was in the middle of studying for my Diploma in Teaching English as a Foreign Language, as well as teaching full time, and the house was a tranquil haven for my tired brain at the end of each busy day. Chris and Rebecca mended fences, built new ones and reconstructed the hen house. We bought hens and took a photograph of the first egg. We planted a vegetable garden. At night, in the intense blackness devoid of city lights, we stood in the garden under a sky crammed with stars, listening to the silence and feeling that we were the luckiest people on earth.

Rebecca explored the quiet lanes and riverbed on Red and persuaded me to start riding so we could explore the neighbourhood together. Not having her natural flair for risk-taking, I was nervous about mounting Red, but eventually I got on him, and she led me around the paddock and out down the road.

'Mum! Relax, will ya! Look at your knuckles. They're *white*!'

Rebecca found someone who practised natural horsemanship to give us lessons. At Darryn's place in Darfield, where he'd built a training arena out of old telegraph poles, Rebecca rode his chestnut quarterhorse, Bug. She said it would be her dream to own a quarterhorse one day. Lace, skittish from the start, threw her off once too often and then one day she threw Natasha off, jumped over the hedge and took off down the road. Rebecca sold her and bought a series of other horses, all more or less crazy. She trained them and sold them on.

She finished the year at Lincoln and started playing ice hockey in town as well as riding. She decided not to return to Lincoln the following year because the equine option in her course was not continuing. Fabiano and Bruno wrote from Brazil and said they'd like to come and visit us in the summer of 1998 so Rebecca decided to put off looking for a job so she could spend the summer with them.

In the meantime Grant and Bart bought an old bomb of a car and Rebecca asked if they could keep it in our garden for a 'short while'. Every weekend the boys came out and tinkered with the car. Rebecca and Natasha rode their horses and threw horse poo over the fence at the boys. One day we all went out to watch Rebecca jumping bareback on Red.

I heard Bart's sharp intake of breath. 'If Becks misses, she's in trouble.'

'Yeah,' from Grant.

But when Rebecca returned there was no sign of the anxiety I'd seen etched on their faces, and they continued to hurl abuse at each other. Rebecca dared the boys to ride bareback. They took up the challenge, turning white, trying to look cool, and complaining it was like sitting on a pile of jelly.

As the weeks passed the car assumed gaudier colours, which they all contributed to, along with rude messages and cartoons from the girls. During the day they charged along the dry riverbed in the car. They found an old wooden bridge on wheels across the river and carved their initials in the side. In the evenings they occasionally scrubbed up and went out to town for a meal or a movie.

Bruno arrived in January and stayed with us for four weeks. During his stay we all went to see *Titanic*. Rebecca waved at a group of young people who were standing watching her in the foyer of the cinema.

'Do you know them?' I asked.

She shook her head.

The next day the phone rang and someone asked to speak to my daughter. I handed Rebecca the phone and when she put it down she laughed and said that the young man she'd waved to had followed her to the car, taken a note of the number plate and had been able to trace our phone number. He'd asked her out.

'What!' I gasped. 'He's probably a psychopath!'

Bruno was highly amused. 'But this is normal in Brazil.'

'Not in New Zealand!' I said.

'Are you going, Rebecca?' he asked.

'No. He's not a horse.'

I breathed a sigh of relief.

In Bruno's fourth week Fabiano arrived for three weeks. The sun blazed almost continuously and the summer was filled with trips around the South Island, the young people swimming with the dolphins in Akaroa, bungee jumping in Hanmer Springs, walking through Broken River Cave in pitch blackness, tramping through the bush, picnics and movies and theatre and music. The swimming pool at home echoed with their laughter.

When Bruno flew back to Brazil, Fabiano had two more weeks. One evening as I was cooking dinner in the kitchen he came to stand beside me. When he didn't say anything I turned to look at him and saw tears in his eyes.

'What's up?'

'Two weeks,' he said. 'I can't believe it! I don't want to go back. I'll be homesick for New Zealand.'

I told him what Marilena had said to me, that we'd always have a home in Brazil. This was true for him, too, I said. He'd always have a home with us here.

Out on a walk he asked me if I thought Bruno was still in love with Rebecca. I told him Bruno had a girlfriend in Brazil. A few days later we went to Willowbank, the wildlife reserve, where we'd arranged to meet Susannah and Mark, Benjamin and Dee. To my surprise I saw Rebecca and Fabiano holding hands. Susannah and Benjamin grinned. Rebecca scowled at them and snatched her hand away.

Just before we left Willowbank I asked her about this development. She grimaced. 'The trouble is, I'm not sure I want it.'

When we got home she went straight to bed while Fabiano stayed up and dreamt about a future in New Zealand with Rebecca. A few days later he told me Rebecca had changed her mind. He spent a lot of time in tears behind the old grey poplar in the garden, singing sad songs across the paddock. After this, the tree became known as Fabiano's Tree. He'd had his whole life planned out, he wept. I reminded him he was four and a half years older than Rebecca and while he may be ready to settle down, she was far from that. He should just think of it as a summer romance and leave with happy memories.

He shook his head. 'No. When I looked at her in the park, the whole world disappeared. There was just me and her. We were surrounded by beautiful flowers and I told her she was the most beautiful flower of all. She's the only girl I've ever truly loved. The only one I'll ever love.'

Before he left New Zealand there appeared to be a reconciliation of sorts. Rebecca was cagey about this, but when we went to Whitecliffs for a walk in the river she began speaking in Portuguese to him and allowed him to hold her hand, perched on a rock, while I took a photo.

Knowing how much she disliked public displays of affection, we were surprised to see her kiss him goodbye at the airport. Benjamin grinned and turned away, knowing better than to incur her wrath by commenting. A couple of days later she phoned Fabiano in Brazil and they corresponded for the next 15 months, but while he remained intensely in love, Rebecca's ardour rapidly cooled.

She started a correspondence course in drawing and cartooning. One day she said she felt so tired she couldn't draw. When she couldn't draw I knew she must be really ill, so I was concerned, but a few days later she sat on the verandah with her two cats and her two ferrets and drew a series of hilarious cartoons. I breathed easily again.

That year she worked on a dairy farm, helped train a racehorse, worked on a sheep farm with a farmer called Kevin, played ice hockey and worked at the ice rink several evenings a week and at weekends, and continued to ride her horse and help other people with theirs. She also took some art courses at the polytechnic, the university and the Arts Centre. We continued to ride together and have lessons with Darryn in Darfield.

Susannah decided it was time to groom some of the tomboyishness out of her sister, which had returned as the Brazilian influence faded away. 'She's so pretty, Mum, but she spends all her time in scruffy jeans, mucking about with animals!' She suggested I pay for a modelling and deportment course for Rebecca's 20th birthday. Only because this suggestion came from the beautiful, elegant sister she so admired did Rebecca agree to do the course.

Although family members were invited to the last day of the course to see the finished results, Rebecca would not allow any of us to attend.

'I'd feel like a dick with you lot watching,' she spluttered.

However, there was a photographer present who took a photograph of her that none of us could recognise.

'Hey, you scrub up pretty good,' said Chris.

That much praise she could accept.


It was a huge achievement for me to go out horse riding with Rebecca around our neighbourhood and down to the river. It was during these rides that she opened up and told me things I'd never known about her, as well as her hopes and dreams for the future. She wanted to travel, possibly to Texas to work on a horse ranch for a while, and to Ireland because she loved Celtic history. She'd also like to go to Brazil again and help David with his riding school. Most of all she wanted to buy her own land in the future and breed horses and have lots of animals. She thought she might like to marry some day and have two children. 'They'd have to be born in the saddle though,' she laughed.

Since her childhood, when she'd clung to me like a limpet, she had astonished me with her beauty, her humour, her daring, her energy, and now her ideas for the future. These tumbled over each other with such rapidity I lost track of them. I was amazed by this girl of ours, and worried constantly that her risk-taking would result in an accident. There was good reason for this. She told me cheerily one day that she'd driven through the level crossing just before the train came through.

'It was pouring with rain and my wipers weren't working that well,' she laughed. 'I saw these red flashing lights, but I must have been away with the fairies because they didn't register until I drove over the crossing. Then I saw the train. *Whoops!*'

She tossed off my lecture with, 'Oh, stop worrying about me. I have nine lives.'

'No, you don't! You're a girl, not a cat!'

# SEVEN

# A death and a birth

In May 1999 we celebrated Rebecca's 21st birthday. I made a birthday cake in the shape of an ice rink and Benjamin and Dee attached coloured pipe cleaners to little figures to make ice hockey sticks for two teams. We decorated the table with some of the model horses Rebecca had collected over the years and we bought her some paints and an easel. In the evening we all went out to the Westpac Centre to a performance of the Chinese Circus. We'd kept this a surprise. As we passed the racetrack I joked that the surprise was to watch a night-time horse race. Susannah and Benjamin gave strangled cries of dismay, but Rebecca beamed, 'Oh *cool!*'

A week later Fabiano returned to New Zealand to do his three months' internship at Christchurch Public Hospital. He lived with us until August. Rebecca was by then playing for two ice hockey teams as well as working at the ice rink. She complained of a sore back. Given all the falls from horses she'd sustained over the years this was not surprising, but an X-ray found nothing amiss, although the doctor recommended a few weeks of physiotherapy.

The pain made her irritable, especially with Fabiano. They went out to parties and movies together, but she made it clear she wasn't interested in him romantically. He was devastated, but joined a choir, made friends at the hospital and tried as best he could to make the most of his time in New Zealand.

In August, the day before he flew back to Brazil, he took Rebecca to the airport and said goodbye as she flew off to play for the national women's ice hockey team in Auckland.

When he returned he went straight to his room in tears. He left a letter under her pillow telling her he'd wait for her and promised he'd come back.

Rebecca was greatly moved by the letter. She was sorry she'd hurt him, but it was because she was not good at dealing with feelings, she said. She couldn't find the right words, so she'd ended up being abrupt with him. This bothered her, but she didn't know what to do about it.

'This always happens to me,' she said. 'I'm interested in someone until they get too interested in me and then, it's like … window-shopping is fun, but I don't want to buy.'

'Well,' I said, 'you're young. You've got all the time in the world.'

'Yeah, but I don't want to get serious with anyone,' she said. 'Guys just slow you down.'

'One day you'll change your mind about that.'

She shook her head. 'Nope. Not me. I've got too much stuff to do.'

Darryn came out to give me a lesson on Red and we all set off down the road towards the river, with Rebecca on Ezra. With no warning, Ezra bucked and Rebecca fell into the road with Ezra's heels kicking out at her head. She rolled away and stood up, concerned more for Ezra than for herself. She got back on him and he immediately bucked her off again. Darryn suggested we go back home and do some work on him in the paddock. Although he said Rebecca shouldn't mount again if she was uncomfortable, she got back in the saddle. She said Ezra either had a sore back or he'd been mistreated at some point in his life.

As we rode home I asked Darryn if he'd ever thought of selling Bug. He said he'd just put him on the market that day, for $4000. This was a great deal more than we'd paid for a horse before. I thought of all the crazy horses Rebecca had ridden. There was a reason they were so cheap. Even Red, she discovered, had a deep, indented scar at the back of his tongue where he'd obviously been tied with wire. Chris agreed with the idea of buying Bug. We rang Darryn to confirm it and went out to tell Rebecca just as she was driving away.

She wound the window down and I said, 'For your next birthday, and all your birthdays and Christmases for the next ten years, we've bought Bug for you.'

Her jaw dropped. For once she was speechless.

When Bug arrived she walked around for days saying, 'I have a *quarterhorse*. I can't *believe* it!'

They formed an instant bond. He followed her around the paddock, nuzzling her hair with his big nose. One day she stood on his bare back while he grazed. 'How many lives do you think you've got left?' I complained.

Her answer was to turn in a complete circle on Bug's back.

At the end of the year she organised her portfolio of artwork and applied to the Art and Design degree course at Christchurch Polytechnic. She said she was really looking forward to doing the course and also wanted to join a drama group.

In November she complained of a pain in her left side. An X-ray showed nothing. The doctor told her to come back if it didn't get better. But her tolerance of pain and discomfort was high. She never mentioned it again and I forgot about it.

She started her Art and Design course in February 2000. We travelled into town every day together. Whenever anyone asked her how her course was going she responded, 'It's *fabulous*! I just go there and *draw* all day!' She was impressed with the talent of some of the other young people on the course and the commitment of the staff. It was the first time she'd ever been in a class where other people were as devoted to drawing as she was and were at least as talented. She also received acknowledgement of her own talent from the staff and other students. She joined a local drama class and performed in a play at the end of the semester.

We were surprised to see her act in a variety of roles, including, to our amusement, a demure young Catholic girl. Once again, she made friends at the class. Her social life was such that she was hardly ever at home. The drama coach asked if any horse riders in the group were interested in auditioning for *Lord of the Rings*. Rebecca thought long and hard about that. In the end she decided to concentrate on getting her degree.

'There'll be other opportunities,' she said.

The phone rang constantly and the voices at the other end asked for Beth, Rohanna, and Rowan among others, and even, occasionally, for Rebecca.

'It's good to change names to suit the occasion,' she said in response to my query. 'So if they ask for Beth, you know that's the riding club; if it's Rohanna, it's drama; if it's …'

The future stretched ahead, endless and exciting, filled with possibilities. She might be an actor. She'd work in design perhaps. Or animation. That would be *cool*. She'd breed horses, of course. Though first there'd be travel. And of course the Spanish Riding School. For now, however, her art course was all-encompassing and she set herself the goal of being the best she could be. She even gave up ice hockey to concentrate on her art. During the whole of 2000 she was happier and more settled than I'd seen her since she was a child.

Benjamin graduated in April. In July, the novel I'd completed in Brazil was launched.

At the launch Rebecca spent the evening taking photographs. I wanted to take one of her, but she'd used up the whole film.

In August, Chris's mother died at the age of 92. The resthome called us. We left immediately and got there an hour later. Momma was lying in her bed with her mouth wide open. It was a shocking sight and before we could react, Susannah arrived. When she saw her grandmother like that she burst into tears. Benjamin arrived a few minutes later and was so horrified he walked straight out of the room, white-faced. We were bewildered and angry that no one had thought to close Momma's mouth. Only Rebecca regarded the situation with her usual equanimity and kissed Momma goodbye.

In October my new horse arrived, a beautiful palomino quarterhorse. Rebecca had chosen him. We should call him Jade, because he was green, she laughed. As he was only three years old she took over his training until he was ready for me to ride. One day he shied at the gate and Rebecca fell off, grazing her elbow. Normally her cuts and bruises healed very quickly. I was puzzled over the coming months that this graze took so long to heal.

In November, she arranged for us to go to a weekend riding clinic Darryn was running at Coleridge Station. She would ride Jade and I could ride Bug. We arrived early on Saturday morning, had lessons on horsemanship for the rest of the morning and in the afternoon went on a trek. Rebecca wanted to gallop up the side of the hill, but she stayed with me at a sedate pace. 'Are you all right, Mum?' she kept asking, 'Are you happy? Are you enjoying yourself?'

In the evening the group of riders gathered, wine glasses in hand, under a star-packed sky, hungry now for the lamb turning on the spit, which was drenching the chill night air with hot, delicious aromas. Talk and laughter weaved in and out of the country-and-western music on the radio and the soft whinnying of the horses in the nearby paddocks. By 11pm I was ready for bed while Rebecca and some of the others stayed up till the early hours.

Our accommodation was a bunkroom with lumpy mattresses and no curtains at the window, so I was glad when the early morning light woke me from a fitful sleep. One or two riders had slept in their horse floats, which Rebecca thought was a great idea. 'I might do that on the next clinic,' she said.

The morning was spent in more lessons and the horses were going so well everyone was reluctant to leave. Darryn said he would run another clinic in January. As Rebecca drove the horse float home she declared it the best weekend ever. When she graduated from her Art and Design course, she said, she'd like to work with Darryn for a bit.

'You want to do so much,' I laughed. 'How are you going to fit it all in?'

'I've got the rest of my life,' she said.

'True.'

That Christmas was our first with our new grandchild. I thought of my own grandmother with her arms held wide as my brother and I rushed into her ample-bosomed embrace. '*Come here, my canny bairns!*' I thought of the stories she'd told me about her growing up. She remembered when the village green was still a pond. It was filled in when a child drowned in it. The pond had been used to duck witches in the Middle Ages, she said. She often spoke of her regret at not having had a proper education, which meant that, though she loved books, she always had to read with a dictionary. Nonetheless, she had a store of stories that kept me intrigued with life 'in the olden days' and she expanded my imagination. What stories would I pass on to my own grandchildren?

Rebecca said she'd be the auntie who'd teach Elliot to ride. 'Susannah can do all the cuddly stuff,' she said. 'That's not really my thing.'

Natasha moved to Australia with her boyfriend, and Rebecca bought Red from her. She was sad to say goodbye to her best friend, but happy that Red was now hers.

Grant and Bart started jobs, found girlfriends, bought proper cars and moved their old bomb back to town and to a wrecker's yard. They talked longingly about the days at Greendale, working on the old car. Bart told us how stressed he'd been with his electronics course and assignments and deadlines. 'Coming out here was like a different world,' he said. 'By the time I went back to town I was ready to take on the load again.' They thought they might like to get another old car and bring it back to Greendale. Do the same sort of thing. One day.

The summer was hot. Rebecca and I rode every day. Over the following weeks she mentioned that she often felt hungry, but could only eat small amounts. She complained that her stomach was bloated even though she didn't eat much. She started exercising more, going for long walks around the neighbourhood to reduce weight. She occasionally mentioned that she couldn't take a full breath, only half-breaths. I suggested she should swim more to open up her chest muscles. We saw the New Year in swimming under the stars.

Darryn ran another riding clinic in January. Rebecca went to this one alone as I was too busy to go. She came back home bursting with stories of Darryn, the horses and the other participants.

'I asked Darryn if I could leave the group and gallop Red bareback up the hill. He said, "Well, it's a bit risky, but what the hell – you've gotta have fun!"' It was *sooooo* cool!'

I rolled my eyes. '*Cats* have nine lives. Not *girls*!'

'You should've gone, Mum. You'd've *loved* it. Promise me you'll go to the next one?'

I promised.

EIGHT

# Diagnosis

'I've had one of those dreams, Mum!' Susannah's voice sounded worried over the phone. 'The old woman again.'

Susannah and I have always dreamt vividly and for many years we've discussed our dreams with each other. These discussions brought hoots of derision from Chris and Rebecca who claimed they never remembered theirs. My dreams were usually connected to whatever I was writing about at the time. Susannah's dreams, however, have sometimes contained a warning element.

Susannah is observant and insightful and has an uncanny ability to understand situations before anyone else around her does. Chris's mother used to say she was 'fey'. Since childhood many of her dreams have involved meeting a woman whose face keeps changing. Sometimes the face is old, sometimes it is young. It is never possible to see which face is the woman's real face as it changes so rapidly. These meetings take place in a round room with many doors and are always very pleasant, with the woman showing Susannah a different door each time, which she can choose to go through if she wants. The dream she now wanted to tell me about, however, was not pleasant.

'I had to climb up to the top of a mountain. When I got there the old woman came out of her house. She invited me inside because she wanted to show me something. But this time I wasn't pleased to see her. I knew that what she had to show me was something I didn't want to see. I got angry with her and ran away.'

'Maybe you've been worried about something?'

'No, it's more than that, Mum. She's never shown me something negative before. I know something bad is going to happen.'

Rebecca began her second year at the Art and Design School. I drove her into town on the first day of the new term in February. She was unusually subdued, and slept in the car, saying she was very tired. I said she couldn't possibly be tired after such a long summer vacation. I looked at her and saw the blue had drained out of her eyes and left them pale grey. This was a sign that she was indeed unwell.

At the end of February she complained of a nagging pain in her side. She turned up in my office one day asking for a Panadol. I urged her to go to the doctor's, but she kept putting it off, saying she was too busy with deadlines for art projects. Her back was also hurting again. A new teacher in my department, Bronwyn, mentioned that she and her husband, Burje, had just returned from Sweden where he'd been a chiropractor. He'd set up a clinic in Christchurch. I told her about Rebecca's back and she urged me to ring him.

Benjamin was offered a job in Wellington and he, Dee and Elliot moved in with us until he could go to Wellington to find a place for them to live. While they were with us, a fantail flew into Rebecca's bedroom one morning. Dee was uneasy and told Benjamin that a fantail in the house was a warning of death.

'Just superstition,' he said.

'If every time a fantail flew in the house somebody died, we'd all be dead by now,' Chris laughed, opening the window to let it out. My concern was only that the bird got free before one of the cats caught it.

At the beginning of March we celebrated Chris's birthday dinner with Rebecca, Susannah and Mark and Dee.

Rebecca said to her sister, 'Susannah, you're *thirty*! Geez! I don't want to be thirty!'

We laughed and told her she'd have no choice.

She said, 'Well, I won't have to worry about that because I won't live till I'm thirty.'

'Thirty's not *that* old, you know!' said Susannah, indignant.

'I know, but I still won't be thirty.'

We asked how she could possibly know that.

She shrugged. 'I just do.'

She started talking about how awful it would be to be kept alive on a life support system. 'Me and Natasha promised each other that if either of us was in an accident and ended up on a life-support system, the other would turn it off.'

She also said she'd hate to be buried and made me promise to cremate her. I told her to stop being so morbid.

'Mum, you must *promise*. I mean it. *Promise!*'

I promised, adding that parents didn't usually bury their children and I hoped I wouldn't have to make that decision as she'd be burying me. Susannah joined in saying that when I died she'd cremate me.

'I couldn't stand the idea of you being in the soil, Mum. I'd scatter your ashes in the air and know you were free.'

'I hadn't thought of it like that,' I said.

Chris said he couldn't care less whether they buried him or cremated him. They could put him on the compost heap for all he cared. 'Once you're dead, you're dead. You don't know anything about it.'

He and Rebecca agreed that organ donation at least gave someone a benefit. They'd both stated in their driver's licences that they'd donate their organs in the event of a car accident. Susannah and I weren't so sure.

Benjamin asked if we could *please* change the subject?

A few nights later I had a dream that Rebecca was lying dead in her bed. I awoke in such panic that I wanted to go to her room to check on her. I lay awake for hours. Next morning I told her about the dream. She rolled her eyes. 'Well, I'm glad you didn't come in and wake me up just for that!'

I made an appointment on 8 March for Rebecca to see Burje about her back and told her she should mention the pain in her side at the same time. We went there on the way from work. Burje was a huge bear of a man with a great sense of humour that appealed to Rebecca. He worked on her back for three hours and with a lot of manipulation and acupuncture, improved the flexibility. When he finished, she stood up and said the pain had gone.

She told him about the pain in her side. He used acupuncture on her abdomen then straightened up, glancing at Bronwyn with a frown.

'You have no stomach energy whatsoever,' he said. 'It could be appendicitis.' He added that he felt her appendix was about to burst and she needed to get to a doctor immediately.

Thinking this was surely an exaggeration, I said I would make an appointment next day as it was now late afternoon and the doctor's surgery would be closed. However,

Burje insisted it was urgent and that I should ring the doctor from his house. I rang the locum at the medical centre in Darfield, rather than double back to our normal GP in Christchurch. She said she would open up the centre as it was after hours.

I was sitting in the waiting room flicking through magazines when the doctor came out and told me she'd found a mass.

'It's probably nothing,' she said. 'Young girls often get ovarian cysts. However, I'd like her to get checked out as soon as possible at Christchurch Women's. The X-ray department will be closed now, but I'll make an appointment for you first thing in the morning.'

At the hospital next day I waited and waited, still expecting to be told there was nothing wrong.

I asked a nurse what was taking so long.

She said, 'Has anyone told you what they found?'

I shook my head.

She hesitated. 'I'd better let a doctor tell you.'

Cold, clammy fear in my belly. The doctor came in and sat down. She said there was a seven-centimetre tumour on Rebecca's ovary and fluid in her abdomen. It was probably benign, she said, but because there was fluid in the abdomen it was best to have a closer look. They would operate that afternoon. My mouth went dry. Rebecca asked if she could watch the operation.

'Believe me, you wouldn't want to,' laughed the doctor. She told me to go back to work and come back after the operation.

I returned to work. Chris went to the hospital and waited. I was in the middle of observing some students in their teaching practice when Chris put his head round the door. He said the doctors wanted to talk to us. He said there was probably nothing to worry about, but in the car I couldn't breathe.

The surgeon came into the room with his registrar, a young woman with bright red lipstick. They looked grim as they sat down. They'd removed one of Rebecca's ovaries, the surgeon said. The operation had been successful and Rebecca was now recovering. I let out my breath. However, there were unusual cells on the outside of the ovary and it had been sent to the lab for tests to determine what they were.

Chris murmured, 'Unusual?'

I looked at the registrar with the red lips, but her eyes were fixed on the floor.

'Is it cancer?' I asked the surgeon, not for one moment believing it could be.

He wouldn't be drawn. He'd been wrong before, he said. It could be any one of a number of things. We could go and see Rebecca in recovery in a short while. Not just yet because she was having difficulty with pain. The Pain Team were trying to get it under control. Then we could see her.

As soon as Rebecca saw me she called out, '*Muuum!*'

I put my arms around her. I wanted to wrap her up and take her home and rewind the film.

She said, 'Where's Dad?'

I said he was on his way.

She said, 'Where's the man with the mop?' and drifted off for a few seconds.

Back in her room, still hanging on to my hand, she told me that when it came time for the operation she was very frightened and when she woke up it hurt a lot. I asked if she'd like me to stay overnight. She nodded, her eyes wide with fear. When she was asleep I made a few phone calls. First I called Susannah and then Benjamin. That phone call is etched deep into his memory. It was the first one he'd received from us since going up to Wellington the previous week to start his new job and his new life. Later that evening two colleagues arrived and waited for me downstairs with a large bunch of flowers. I was already crying when I saw them. They hugged me and their own tears started flowing.

The two doctors visited again in the morning. They didn't want to talk to us until Rebecca woke up. Patient confidentiality. I insisted they tell me. Well, this was most irregular not to tell the patient first, but, well, yes, they'd found some malignant cells. Although the form of cancer was very rare – he saw only one case per year in the whole of the South Island – it was treatable with a very good chance of cure in young women. They would arrange further tests the following week.

Within seconds the world stopped making sense. I could taste blood in my mouth. The doctor's face was expressionless. The young woman with the red lipstick still looked at the floor. They wanted to go and tell Rebecca now. I told them to wait until she'd recovered, but they said it was best for her recovery to hear the news immediately then she could deal with it.

As soon as Rebecca opened her eyes they said, 'We found some malignant cells on your ovary. It *is* cancer.'

Her eyes filled with tears. She glanced at me. I touched her hand, but she pulled it away.

The doctor asked, 'Do you have any questions?'

She shook her head.

They left.

I followed and asked to speak in private to the doctor. He took me into a room.

'Is she going to die?'

He shrugged. 'She's young and strong. She has a better chance because of that.'

I talked about her talents, her art, her horse riding, her ice hockey. What was happening now simply couldn't be true. She was young and strong and healthy. How could she possibly have *cancer*? Would it have made any difference if we'd noticed six months ago? He said if we'd noticed six months ago or in six months time it wouldn't have made any difference to the outcome.

Outcome? What did he mean by outcome? When would she need to start chemotherapy?

Again he shrugged. We'd have to talk to the oncologist about that. Some tumours didn't respond to chemotherapy, he said, so the oncologist may want to discuss quality of life. In any case they'd let her recover from this first. In six weeks he'd organise an appointment with the oncologist.

Finally, exasperated by my questions and no doubt exhausted, he shook his head, tears in his eyes. 'Please. Don't do this to me. I can't answer you because I don't know.'

Shocked, I stood up.

He said he was sorry, but he had to go. Would I like to speak to a counsellor?

I nodded.

The hospital chaplain arrived. She was kind, gentle. She used words like journey, travelling together. It wasn't her fault, but I knew I wouldn't ask to see her again.

That night I phoned my brother in England, but he was out. I doubted I could say the words anyway. Instead I wrote him a letter and posted it. I had an overwhelming need for my mother, but she'd been dead 17 years.

The next day on the way to the hospital we drove past a cemetery. Feeling sick to my stomach, I turned my head away from it. Next we passed Riccarton Riding Club. Young girls riding their horses. The sky above them shining blue.

Over the next week doctors came and went. They were still trying to get information on the tumour before they could recommend treatment. The results were inconclusive. Some tumours were benign, but a couple were malignant. Rebecca would have to have a CT scan of her whole body and intestines the following week. The doctor who told us this could give little more information. 'I wish you luck,' she said brusquely. 'That's all I can say.'

The nurses were better. They had more time to listen and they hugged me and joked with Rebecca. They encouraged me to talk to them. I expressed disbelief over and over again.

One of the nurses said, 'She's very sick.'

I said, 'But no, that's not right. She's one of the healthiest people I know.'

She patted my arm.

Grant and Bart came every day. I was deeply impressed by their ability to talk about the situation and keep Rebecca earthed. She told me she'd been dreaming of Bruno and Fabiano and the summer they'd all spent together. She wished she could see them again.

Susannah had a dream where Rebecca was surrounded by many women. One of them spoke to Susannah and explained they were healers. She showed Susannah some stones. Some had the symbol of the crab on them. Some were crab fossils. I asked if she knew the crab was the symbol for cancer. No, she didn't. She remembered she'd found a large crab fossil on Glenfarrick Beach near Christchurch, many years before. A couple of weeks before the cancer was diagnosed Rebecca had asked us to go to Glenfarrick with her so she could find some fossils for herself. Her keen eyes had found many, including a spectacular crab.

I dreamt that my cousin, Maurice, with whom I'd grown up and who had died of colon cancer, came to see me. Rebecca had been 12 when he died. As she grew up I noticed she had a resemblance to him and I hoped that her resemblance was not too close. In the dream I told him how angry I was that my child had cancer at the age of 22. He simply smiled at me and asked me to dance with him.

We began exploring alternative therapies that could be used in conjunction with chemotherapy. Our friend Darina said she would give Rebecca reiki. Burje said he would see Rebecca for continued acupuncture treatments. He gave me the name of the best homeopathic practitioner in New Zealand and I phoned this man to arrange treatment.

The results came back. There was no sign of cancer elsewhere in her body, but the primary site could not be identified. They believed the tumour originated in the intestines, that it was glandular and had probably been present from birth. Although they'd removed her right ovary there were small dots of cancer on her left ovary and peritoneum, the lining of the abdominal cavity. The tumour was a poorly differentiated mucinous adenocarcinoma with signet cells. I looked it up on the Internet.

This tumour was so rare it accounted for only 0.04 per cent of all cancers and usually attacked the 60+ age group. This was a very aggressive cancer that spread extremely quickly. Almost no research had been done on it and only 70 cases had been reported in the USA between 1973 and 1998. Signet cell involvement had the worst prognosis. Most websites gave survival statistics for various types of cancer, but not for this one. Finally I found one that gave a five-year survival rate of 20 per cent.

I climbed into bed beside Chris.

'It's after midnight,' he murmured sleepily. 'What've you been doing?'

'Internet stuff.'

'Is that a good idea?'

'I want to find out, but there isn't much information. According to one website Rebecca could be dead within three months.'

We lay in silence. However, as I knew this statistic could not possibly be true and could not possibly include Rebecca, I fell asleep. Chris told me in the morning there had been no more sleep for him that night.

Not until 2008 did I find a website with detailed information on the kind of cancer Rebecca had, as well as the most successful treatment and many useful links. The woman who'd compiled this information, an American called Carolyn Langlie-Lesnik, had been diagnosed in the same month and year as Rebecca. Although several doctors had told her there was no chance for her survival, she persisted with her research and tracked down a surgeon at the Memorial Sloan-Kettering Cancer Center in New York City who agreed to treat her. Six years later she was still alive and she decided to use her survival as a way to pass on to others the information that hadn't been available to her when she needed it.

Our GP, Peter Law, rang. We'd known him since coming to New Zealand from England 30 years before. When I was pregnant with Rebecca I gave him Frederick Leboyer's book *Birth Without Violence* and told him this was how I wanted the birth to go. He said he liked the book and he'd do what he could to ensure the birth was the way I wanted. Unfortunately, when I went into labour he was away on holiday with his family, so he missed the birth, to his great regret.

When he rang his first words were, 'This should never have happened. This is the wrong age group. She should never have got cancer in this age group.'

But she did.

# NINE

# The scent of summer grass

Rebecca was discharged at the end of the week. She needed six weeks of recovery, the doctors said, before they could start chemotherapy.

When we got home she said, 'I want to get out of this bloody nightie. And I don't want to hear the word cancer mentioned again. Okay?'

Okay.

For the first fortnight she walked about with difficulty because of the pain in her side, then gradually this pain subsided and she said it felt good to be free of pain for the first time in months. I asked her why she hadn't told me it had been going on for months and she said she'd just assumed it would go away eventually.

As paper, wood shavings, glue and paint once again began to cover her bedroom floor, her desk, and then spread out to the living room, I knew I could believe she was getting better. She drew an oil pastel sketch of an Indian girl leading a horse. I marvelled at the luminous quality of the skin and asked her how she achieved it. As she explained, I sat beside her and drew a face in pink pastel. We both burst out laughing. She didn't want to discuss her diagnosis except to say that when she'd originally felt the pain in her side the thought it might be cancer crossed her mind and she imagined what she'd say to her friends.

After four weeks she started to run again and the day she jumped over the paddock gate I felt I could breathe freely. At the end of six weeks we went back to the hospital for her check-up. The surgeon who'd taken out her ovary and given her the cancer diagnosis rubbed his eyes wearily when we entered the room. He asked Rebecca how she was, but didn't examine the site of the surgery until I told him it appeared infected.

'Ah yes, I suppose I should look at it,' he said.

He agreed it was infected and prescribed antibiotics. I asked if the slow healing was due to an infection or to cancer.

'That's a good question,' he said. 'I don't know.' He said he would refer Rebecca to an oncologist.

At the beginning of April, Chris, Rebecca and I sat in the oncologist's waiting room. Pink walls and grey carpet. Volunteers with soft smiles offering cups of tea to grey-faced, elderly women in turbans with missing eyebrows and eyelashes. A frenetic radio voice gabbled that something was only $99.95. A woman on reception droned, 'So I said to him, I says "Yer've gotta be kidding?" But sod it all, they're welcome to each other, that's all I can say, 'cos when all's said and done ...' I read a whole page of the *Woman's Weekly* and had no idea what I'd just read. Chris sat in silence. Rebecca stared at the floor.

A nurse ushered us into the oncologist's office. When I shook his hand I realised my palms were damp. He asked Rebecca how she was feeling. She said she was fine. He said he would be designing her programme of chemotherapy and would be seeing her regularly during her treatment.

Then he sighed and said, 'This is unlikely to cure you. What it *will* do is give you time.'

The three of us were poleaxed into silence.

Rebecca was the first to break it. 'You mean this won't cure it?'

He sighed again. 'Unfortunately, no. Regrettably, this disease will shorten your life. I'm sorry. If you want to ask me any questions I'll answer them honestly.'

We sat stunned.

He asked if we'd like a cup of tea.

I shook my head. Chris and Rebecca walked back to the waiting room. I waited till they were out of earshot and told him not to talk like that again in front of Rebecca. We, our whole family, were committed to beating this disease.

He looked shocked. 'No one has told you this before?'

'No.'

Another sigh. He'd assumed, he said, that I already knew the prognosis. He was so sorry it had been broken to us like this. Was I sure no one had said this before? Was I absolutely sure this hadn't been discussed with us?

No, it had not. And we didn't want to hear it again. What we wanted was for him to cure her.

He promised he'd do his best.

I drove Rebecca home. Chris went back to work. Later that night in the warmth and darkness of our own bed, whispering so Rebecca couldn't hear, he told me he'd locked himself in his office and screamed.

When we got home Rebecca went into my study and burst into tears. I knelt beside her and reminded her of all the difficult horses she'd trained; how she'd ridden bareback up steep hills; how she'd played ice hockey, one of the most dangerous sports in the world; how she'd never turned her back on danger or challenge. Did she want to give up now? Or did she want to do her best to beat this disease?

She nodded through her tears.

Then that's what we'd all commit ourselves to doing. Okay?

Okay.

Tests and more tests. The doctors believed the cancer had originated in the intestines and had been resolved by Rebecca's immune system. But not before it had spread to her abdomen. At the end of April she had two rounds of chemotherapy in one week and would have six more, a combination of leucovorin and fluorouracil. This made her sick, tired and depressed. She was also on a regime of homeopathic medicine, herbs, acupuncture and reiki. As the news spread, our friends around the world phoned and wrote to say they were praying for her.

Chris went with her to the chemotherapy sessions. Our friend Helen, a doctor in the USA, sent me the name of a friend of hers in Christchurch who'd been diagnosed with ovarian cancer and was in remission. I contacted this woman and met her for coffee. She told me she worked in the hospital, so it would be easy for her to visit Rebecca and support her through the chemotherapy sessions, and she did so. She gave me a soft hat she'd worn in bed when all her hair fell out. She said Rebecca would find it useful.

A few days after the first round of chemotherapy Rebecca started to feel better and went for a riding lesson with Darryn. I rode with her to the river twice in the week following. All the time I was riding I was aware of the fast beating of my heart. I wondered how long it had been beating at this speed. It seemed to be permanently over-wound.

After dinner at Susannah's one evening in early April, Rebecca announced she had a surprise for me. She drove me to the Westpac Centre and wouldn't say where we were going.

'You'll love it, Mum,' she laughed. 'That's all I'm saying. You'll just have to wait and see!'

It turned out she'd bought tickets for the Spanish Riding School performance. When I realised this I told her I'd seen it advertised months ago and had intended to buy tickets for us both, but she'd obviously been more on the ball than I had. She was delighted with my pleasure. I, however, was more touched that she'd contrived such a surprise and with her comment, 'I thought you needed something to take your mind off this bloody cancer!'

This was the first time she'd been in a public place since her operation. As we watched the performances and admired the magnificent white horses, it was easy to pretend our world was normal again. We saw the sister of a girl Rebecca had stabled her horse with before we went to Brazil. We'd seen this girl at a riding clinic earlier in the year and at that time we'd chatted to her about breeds of horses, riding techniques and feeding regimes. Now, when I pointed the girl out, Rebecca shook her head. No, she didn't want to talk to her. In the interval she spoke of her plans to go to the Spanish Riding School one day and how she'd like to train a white horse.

It was April 5, 2001. A year and a day before she died.

Over the next weeks she began eating again and running around the paddocks and jumping over all the gates. She said the pain in her abdomen had disappeared and she felt that the cancer had gone. However, the effects of the ongoing chemotherapy left her sick and weak and she didn't feel like painting or drawing. I wouldn't allow myself to feel confident until she did.

She suggested we go and see a Clydesdale/thoroughbred foal she'd seen advertised at a station in the Lees Valley. I reminded her she already had four horses.

She nodded. 'I know. But this is just to look at.'

We followed the breeder's instructions to wait on the other side of the river and toot our horn. As we waited for her to drive down in her truck Rebecca looked around at the hills and wide open spaces and said, 'This is exactly the kind of life I want. I want to live somewhere like this and breed horses and have dozens of cats. I'd like all sorts of animals actually.'

'And I'll come and live with you when I'm old and decrepit.'

'Of course you will!' she said with conviction.

The breeder took us to see the mares and the Clydesdale stallion and finally the five foals, all five months old. Rebecca fell in love with a deep chestnut filly and asked if she could have it.

I laughed. 'So this was just to look at, was it?'

She said, 'I know, but it would help me. A new life. Something for me to focus on.'

We arranged for it to be delivered the following week. As we sat with a cup of tea in the breeder's kitchen I asked if she felt afraid of her isolation. What happened if someone fell sick? She agreed it was a problem. Someone had had a heart attack there and died. Just the previous week there'd been a horse trek on the hills. The horse had slipped and fallen over a steep ridge. Horse and rider died.

'How terrible,' I gasped.

Rebecca disagreed. 'Exactly how I'd like to go. Doing what I love.'

I talked to Peter Law, our GP. He said when he'd seen Rebecca the day before it was hard to believe she was sick as she looked so healthy. He added she was completely atypical in this situation; it was so rare as to be almost impossible in her age group; she had no symptoms and looked so healthy and the primary tumour had apparently disappeared. He said none of it made any sense, but he believed a positive outcome was a strong possibility.

Rebecca picked up her art projects from her tutors and decided to work on them at home over the three weeks of the Easter holiday. However, as the chemo sessions progressed she became progressively more miserable, tired and nauseous. For the first time since the sessions began, she cried. She said she was hungry, but couldn't eat. She was thirsty, but couldn't drink. In addition, the pain in her abdomen was back. Chris and I held her and let her cry all she wanted. After that she was able to eat a little and drank three glasses of juice. I talked to her and said she didn't have to try to be brave over this disease. She just wanted to be held. When she came home after the final session she went straight to bed and slept all afternoon.

Two months earlier life had been so simple. I enjoyed my teaching, my writing, riding with Rebecca, gardening, working on house projects, planning for the future. Now cancer took all my time and energy. Rebecca, however, did not want to read about cancer or even discuss it. I spent hours on the internet. I continued teaching because it helped me stay grounded, but I no longer had any time, energy or desire to write. I could no longer remember my dreams. Chris took three months leave of absence from his lecturing, going into the office only to do some admin tasks. His colleagues filled the gaps he left and no one made any demands on him, something he says he'll never forget.

Marilia and Sebastião, our friends in Brazil, told us about a herbal medicine made by a 90-year-old pharmacist and a group called Caminho da Luz which specialised in treating cancer. She asked me to send Rebecca's lab reports for her to have translated by a doctor there and have the medicine made up. However, New Zealand Post would not agree to send it, so Sebastião investigated going through the New Zealand Consulate in São Paulo.

The new foal arrived on 26 April. Rebecca and I leaned over the gate to the paddock and the foal came and stood between us. The sky was blue with white, wispy clouds. There was no wind, and no sound but the foal's breathing. Rebecca was grinning from ear to ear as she talked about her plans for training this foal. She'd be great for long treks, she enthused. The foal had the same colouring as Cristiane, so Rebecca wanted to incorporate Cristy's name and came up with Kit Silver.

Later that afternoon Kit jumped a fence and ran down the road. We drove after her and blocked the road. Rebecca stood waiting a little distance away till the foal decided to approach her. She then slipped the halter over Kit's head and led her back home. After that, Jade, my young quarterhorse, took Kit under his wing, but Red and Bug kept chasing and biting her so we put those two in a separate paddock till they got used to the sight and smell of her.

Rebecca went out into the paddock every day to work with Kit, grooming her and talking to her. Rebecca's eyes were bright and her cheeks were pink. It was impossible to believe she wasn't in the best of health. The weekend after Kit arrived we went on a trek with our riding group, to Kowhai Bush. Rebecca rode Jade and I rode Bug. At the end of the trek we sat in the warm grass eating our picnic, chatting to the other women. The smell of sweet summer grass is the smell I always associate with Rebecca. The smell of sun-saturated warmth and the outdoors. She said she felt strong and energetic, had no pain and she knew the cancer was going away. I believed her, but my heart still ticked like an overwound clock.

The next cycle of chemotherapy was scheduled for 7 May but Rebecca's white blood count was still too low, so it was postponed for another week. When we left the office she cried. She hated seeing the oncologist, she said, and the whole situation depressed her. She also said she didn't want to go back to her art course. I said if she just stayed at home she'd have too much time to focus on the illness and the chemo. Being with her friends and painting every day would help keep her focused on other things.

A few days after this she came to see me in my office and asked me to go to the library with her to pick up some books she'd chosen. These were heavy tomes on horses and the different colours of their coats, manes and tails. At home she referred to the books to paint a model horse she'd had since childhood. From time to time she'd painted this horse with whatever colour was her favourite of the moment. Now she painted it palomino gold. She also worked on a project for her art course. This involved making a scaffold where three clay racehorses stood with nooses around their necks. This was, she said, meant to represent the racing industry and the healthy young horses which were destroyed simply because they'd failed to win a race.

Benjamin, Dee and Elliot came to stay with us and we had a family dinner to celebrate Rebecca's 23rd birthday on 9 May. My and Chris's gift to her was an oiled riding coat and I took a photo of Susannah, Benjamin and Rebecca standing together, Rebecca in her new coat, smiling, her blonde hair pulled back in a ponytail. There was no sign on the photo of the thinning parting we'd noticed two weeks after the first chemotherapy treatment. She enjoyed the evening and the time with her brother and sister so much that her spirits lifted. After they left she began painting again and worked for six hours on a project.

She called in to see Kevin, the farmer she'd worked for the previous year. He was in his seventies and Rebecca loved his company and his sense of humour. When she returned home I asked if she'd had a good day.

'I've had a *great* day,' she grinned.

Kevin had taken her to the races and then to the pub where they'd met some of his friends. She often told me that despite his wish to present a tough, crusty exterior she knew he was a softie. The fact he'd kept his old race horse in retirement on his farm endeared him to her enormously. At the end of the year she dismantled her scaffold and gave him one of the clay horses for Christmas with the name of his own racehorse inscribed. When Chris and I visited him a few months after Rebecca's death, he brought this little clay horse out to show us. Though he professed not to be religious, I noticed he had a rosary wound around it.

'I'll never forget the day she was ploughin' one of the paddocks,' he said. 'Every line was straight except for the middle of the paddock where she'd gone round in a circle. I asked her what the hell she'd been doin' and she said there was a bird sittin' on a nest and she didn't have the heart to disturb it!' And he roared with laughter. Following the laughter he shook his head and dashed his hand across his eyes. 'Then come the day she told me she didn't want to be a farmer. "I hate sheep," she said, "and I hate tractors". And I says to her, "Well whaddya want to do?" and she says, "I'm goin' to apply to art school." And I told her I was glad to hear it 'cos she was too much of a lady and far too pretty to be doin' farmin'. And she gives me one of them looks of hers!' He laughed again. 'Yer know the one?'

Yes, we did.

I told him how much Rebecca had enjoyed working for him and how much she'd loved his humour.

Alma, Kevin's wife, rolled her eyes. 'She was the only one that did! He's not the easiest person to get on with!'

Kevin responded by telling the story of the time he and Rebecca had travelled to the West Coast with a racehorse and they'd stayed with his brother and his wife. 'They loved her to bits. She got on real well with old people.' He shook his head. 'I think of her every day. I love her as much as I do my own granddaughters. I look at this little horse and the paintin' she gave me and I pray for her. God love us, she shouldn't have got cancer. Not *her*.'


The oncologist rang. I could hear the excitement in his voice.

'The cancer markers are decreasing. We have a tumour that responds to chemo-therapy!'

When I told Rebecca she grinned. 'I know. It's no longer in my body.'

Burje continued to give her regular acupuncture treatments and firmly refused to accept payment from us. He shook his large head, with its thatch of dark hair, from side to side. If I mentioned it again he'd be gravely offended. To Rebecca he said, 'My payment will be when you walk in here two years from now and give me a big hug.'

He also told her not to have chemotherapy as all her white blood cells would be destroyed and the slightest infection could kill her. Nor should she use other forms of medication, whether orthodox or alternative, as it would negate the effects of his treat-ment. Chris and I had a meeting with him where we insisted he respect our decision to leave no stone unturned when it came to deciding what treatments we'd pursue and that he must not encourage Rebecca to stop chemotherapy. Although he was strongly opinion-ated I couldn't fault his genuine desire to help Rebecca. There was no doubt she benefited from his great sense of humour and his belief that he could make her better. I didn't want to fall out with him and I was glad that he agreed to accept our decision.

The oncologist showed us the results of Rebecca's blood tests. Before the chemo started, the cancer markers, the CA 125, had shown a level of 108. With a big smile on his face he told us it was now 68. Normal was 65. It seemed to be an affirmation for Rebecca that she was right about the cancer disappearing. I slept through the night for the first time in two months.

My friend Darina gave Rebecca a reiki treatment, with another friend, Penny.

After the treatment Rebecca sat up and said, 'Mum, who's Sarah McQuillan?'

'Your great-grandfather's sister. Why?'

'She was here. I asked her three times if I would live and she said yes. Each time I asked her she said YES really loud.'

I burst into tears. So did Darina and Penny.

On 14 May Chris took her in for her second round of chemo. The oncologist called him and said the rest of her chemo that week had been cancelled. They'd just received the latest results of the tests on her ovary. The conclusion was that although they still hadn't located the primary tumour, they believed now that the cancer had originated in the ovary and not the gastro-intestinal tract. 'She's well. She's healthy. She isn't wasting away. She shows none of the symptoms of GI cancer,' he said. The new type of chemo they would give her wouldn't be so aggressive. It would be one day every three weeks instead of five days every month. With this new treatment she had a 70 per cent chance of survival. She might need more surgery to remove as much of the cancer as possible. We were buoyed with hope and optimism. When we returned home Rebecca took Bug out for a ride.

Next day we saw the surgeon who'd originally operated on Rebecca. When we walked into his room our hopes rapidly sank. He said that the pathologists had been so certain that the cancer had originated in the GI tract that they hadn't sent the ovary to Australia for further tests as they'd planned. However, they had run more tests on it and those tests showed a high probability of the cancer having originated in the ovary. They then decided to send it to Australia for another opinion and those tests would be back in a week or two. He said the reason they'd run further tests was because the whole situation was atypical of GI tract cancer. Rebecca's young age, the fact her CA 125 was not very elevated and the fact she appeared to be so healthy, whereas they would have expected her to be very sick by now, meant that they were going to treat the cancer as ovarian, which would mean a different chemo. While it didn't have the side effects of the previous chemo it would make all her hair fall out. She'd suffer from diarrhoea and vomiting. She'd also need a total hysterectomy and possibly some of her bowel removed. If that happened she'd have a temporary colostomy to allow the bowel to heal. The chemo would deal with the rest of the cancer that might be left behind. With ovarian cancer there was an 80 per cent chance of remission. But only 30 per cent with GI cancer.

I felt all the blood drain from my head and I crumpled to the floor. The doctor asked the nurse to take me into the waiting room. Rebecca was in tears. When I went back into the room the doctor was in tears too. He said the prognosis was much better with ovarian cancer and he wanted to give her the best possible chance of recovery. He also told her how much he respected her bravery.

Outside, Rebecca insisted on driving me home. 'You're in no state to drive!' she said. She also added that she didn't want to see that surgeon again because every time she saw him he managed to extinguish any spark of hope and optimism she had. 'I always feel really good till I see him,' she said. We stopped off at Burje's where he gave me acupuncture to treat shock and to Rebecca to boost her immune system.

When we got home she went into my study and cried. She said, 'With my luck I'll be in the 20 per cent who *don't* go into remission, so it's not worth going through that treatment.'

I reminded her how her courage had seen her through difficult times; how everyone who met her and got to know her was impressed by her courage and determination; how people she met at riding clinics, whom she couldn't remember meeting before, still recounted the tales of seeing her cantering bareback up and down steep hills on a six-hour trek she'd gone on the previous year, when no one else would ride those hills, even in a saddle.

'Do you remember how Red decided to take off at a gallop one day? Through intersections? Zigzagging across the road? Were you scared then?'

She shook her head. No, because she knew he'd run out of steam in the end and in the meantime she had the skills to know how to stay on his back.

'Exactly. Because you had the strength, determination, courage and willpower to stay on what could've been a very dangerous ride. Those same characteristics let you play national level ice hockey, gained you entrance to a highly competitive Art and Design course, and allowed you, a normally shy person, to join a drama group and act in a play in public. These characteristics will let you achieve anything you set your mind to. If you believe in yourself then nothing can beat you, not even cancer.'

She listened. And agreed to go through with the treatment. She would try to finish the last five weeks of the semester at Art School and then take the rest of the year off to concentrate on her recovery. She asked me to shave off all her hair before it fell out. That way it would be her decision and a way of taking back some control of her life, she said. She rang Bart and Grant and they said they would shave their heads too. Natasha rang and said she was coming back to New Zealand in November for a holiday. All the chemo would be finished by then. If she was well enough, Rebecca thought she might go to Australia for a holiday with Natasha.

That weekend we all felt a little better. Rebecca went on a trek with her riding club. I stayed home to finish a short story called *The Red Bandanna*, based on Rebecca's experiences on David's farm in Brazil when she was training Cristiane. I read her the story. She listened with her eyes closed, smiling at the memories. The story was broadcast on National Radio 18 months afterwards, too late for Rebecca to hear it.

We met the oncologist and the surgeon the following week. They'd just received the results of the tests on Rebecca's ovary from Australia. The results still leaned towards ovarian cancer, but weren't conclusive, and more tests were going to be done that week. However, as the leaning was towards ovarian cancer they wanted to start treating it as that. They would give a combination of Taxol and Carboplatin. Rebecca would stay in hospital for three hours. Three weeks later the second dose would be given and two weeks after that her CA 125 level would be looked at and scans done. If she was responding to the chemo then the conclusion about the cancer being ovarian would be confirmed and surgery would follow. They explained they wanted to cover all bases to give Rebecca the best possible chance of a cure. They said the drugs had recently been tested in a clinical trial and had very encouraging results. They believed these were the best drugs available.

And so the months from May to September passed. Rebecca and I rode along the riverbanks. She painted, and tended her horses. She asked me to write a letter to the surgeon saying she didn't want to see him any more. His rather terse reply arrived a few days later. He certainly had no intention of taking away Rebecca's hope, he wrote, but neither would he give her false hope. I wrote again saying it was in Rebecca's best interests to discontinue appointments with him. There was no reply.

In Susannah's house I cut off Rebecca's beautiful long blonde hair. I held it to my cheek and said I wanted to keep some of it, but she insisted I throw it away. Then I used the shaver. When the job was finished she looked stunning with her bright blue eyes, soft clear skin and fine bones.

'Oh Rebecca, it really suits you,' Susannah said.

'Yeah? Let's have a look.'

After seeing Anna-Marie's shaved head in Brazil she'd been determined to shave her own. I'd persuaded her to delay it until after Susannah's wedding. A bald bridesmaid? No! When we returned to New Zealand she dyed her hair pink and later green, but to my relief forgot about shaving it off. As she stared at herself in the mirror I reminded her she'd finally got her wish. She laughed, pleased with the result.

When Chris arrived I persuaded him to let me trim his hair. The result was a lopsided mess and he was not at all happy, but Susannah, Rebecca and I couldn't stop laughing. Benjamin shaved his own head in support and sent a photo to Rebecca. They looked like twins now, as they'd done when they were little.

In the wig-maker's fitting room Rebecca decided on a long, black wig like Xena the Warrior Princess, her favourite TV programme. She wore it to a friend's 21st party. A few weeks later she said it was too hot to wear, so we went back and got a short blonde wig. She wore that to Art School, but at home, missing the heaviness of hair trailing behind her neck, she tied a scarf around her head.

On her first visit to the oncologist after the new chemotherapy treatment she'd been grey-faced and sullen. His eyes had filled with tears at the sight of her. On our next visit she had make-up on and her blonde wig. His jaw dropped. 'You look like a different girl!'

Peter Law, our GP, joked that the only thing wrong with her was that she had cancer. She laughed and agreed.

In the middle of July a CT scan showed that the widely diffused strands of malignancy in her abdomen and pelvis had disappeared and had localised to one six-centimetre mass behind her uterus. In addition to the improved clinical signs, Rebecca was full of energy and looked well. Even though her blood count was low, she didn't catch the flu that both Chris and I caught. Five days after her third session of Taxol she took Red and Bug to a riding event. It was the first time she'd competed in seven years, but she won five out of the six events she entered and was placed second in the sixth. The oncologist shook his head in disbelief. She passed all her exams at the end of the first semester and finished all her art projects. The only problems appeared to be connected with the side effects of the chemo. She was still strong in the belief she'd recover completely.

Surgery was scheduled then postponed when her blood test showed her CEA (a type of protein molelcule associated with certain tumours) had elevated from 6.3 to 10.9. Normal was 2. Another test was arranged and if it was still elevated she would revert to the previous chemo.

Rebecca finished training Jade. She was also leasing a horse from a girl in the neighbourhood because he was a good jumper and she wanted to do some show jumping. She'd arranged with Mark's sister, Melanie, to take her young filly, Poppy, to train it, and she enjoyed this so much she said she'd like to breed horses if only we had more land. We arranged to buy a further six acres of land from the farmer whose paddocks adjoined ours. He procrastinated so much over the sale that having more land came too late for it to be of any use and after Rebecca died we cancelled the agreement.

On a freezing cold winter's night in July, the hot water tank burst, flooding the spare bedroom. Tanks were bursting all over the South Island because of the unusually cold temperatures. We had no hot water for three weeks while we waited for a new tank to be made so we had to boil up hot water in the kettle every night to fill the bath. When finally the new tank was installed, it felt luxurious being able to have hot showers and baths again. I reflected on how much we took for granted.

At the end of July we lit the fire and Rebecca persuaded me to watch the video, *Gladiator*. I agreed on condition she told me when the gory bits were coming up, so I could close my eyes. At the end of the film Maximus, alias Russell Crowe, lay dying. The haunting music, the rain rattling on the iron roof of our house and the dark sky outside, exacerbated my sense of gloom, which the crackling logs in our potbelly stove did nothing to dissipate. Tears ran down my face.

Rebecca saw this and laughed. 'Mum, there's nothing to cry about. He's reunited with his wife and child again. See, he looks happy.'

I looked up to see a restored gladiator spirit running in slow motion to greet his murdered family. Deep in my belly there was a hollow pain. I felt very afraid. For seven years afterwards I was unable to listen to that music.

Fabiano continued to write to us daily. He was involved in his own drama in Brazil where he was trying to improve his father's run-down farm and bring it up to a productive state again. This met with opposition from his father's mistress whom Fabiano was in the process of trying to oust. He was also trying to decide if he would pursue general surgery or psychiatry as a speciality. Bruno, now married to his girlfriend, Andréia, also wrote. Occasionally Rebecca wrote back to them.

The latest blood test results showed the CEA had elevated from 10.9 to 40 and the CA 125 from 31 to 70. The oncologist said he didn't know why that had happened, but it could have been caused by the disintegration of the tumour and the consequent release of fluid into the body. That would be the most positive reason, he said, but we also had to face the fact that the disease might be progressing and the Taxol and Carboplatin were failing to control it. With that possibility in mind, he decided to change the chemo back to leucovorin and fluorouracil. Rebecca asked him if he was now thinking the tumour could be GI rather than ovarian and he said it could be. However the lab had just run a third test on the tumour and the results were still inconclusive. He said her general appearance and health were not indicative of a GI tumour and as long as she looked well that was the best indicator of what was going on. There would be another CT scan and blood tests at the end of the month and they would review the whole case again. If the tumour was GI in origin they wouldn't operate because it wouldn't help her chances of survival which would only be 30 per cent. If the tumour was ovarian they would operate and she had an 80 per cent chance of going into remission. He ended by saying the chance of someone as young as Rebecca getting this type of cancer was one in a million. I had always known she was a girl in a million. But not like this.

Rebecca now admitted that just before she'd got the results of the blood test she'd had a bad pain in her abdomen for three days and it prevented her from sleeping. She was very upset at the thought of going back to the previous chemo which had made her so sick and she went for a long ride by herself. She found an abandoned lamb in a ditch and brought it home to look after. I told her she'd have no time and energy to raise this lamb, so she should take it back to the farmer.

She stood still, chewing her nails for a moment. 'I hate this bloody cancer!' she sobbed. 'I've lost all my hair. I can't do anything I want. I can't even look after a lamb!'

I pulled her into my arms on the sofa and she cried tears of rage and frustration. When her tears subsided, she talked about all the abandoned lambs she'd found and raised since we'd come to Greendale and I reminded her of the day she'd slung one over Bug's shoulder and rode down the drive of a neighbouring farm. The farmer had looked up, scratched his head and said, 'Now I've seen everything!'

Rebecca remembered the dying lambs she'd brought home from Kevin's farm. 'I knew they were dying. Once you hear that cry you never forget it,' she said. 'But there was no way I could just leave them there in the snow.' Instead they died in our living room. She reminded me of the time one had seemed to rally and then lay down and died. I wouldn't believe it had died and kept trying to nurse it back to health. 'You're such an optimist, Mum!' she laughed.

The day after the first round of leucovorin and fluorouracil I came home to find her in bed, grey-faced, unable to move or speak. Burje asked her to come in every day that week so he could help her overcome these side effects. The following day I came home expecting to find her vomiting and ill again, but to my amazement I saw her running about in the paddocks, pulling electric fences out of the ground. She'd trimmed the fleece around our Angora goat's face. There was no nausea, no exhaustion. She slept well and ate well. We couldn't believe it. She visited Burje every day after her chemo session. She said she always felt terrible when she arrived and fine after an hour and a half of acupuncture. The homeopath sent her some new medicine and she continued to have reiki from Darina.

When we'd originally told Benjamin about the cancer diagnosis he was distraught, especially because he'd just moved to Wellington a week before. He wanted to give up his job and come back home, but when he realised his sister wasn't going to die he calmed down. He phoned me now and said that we'd been through crises before, but had always been able to resolve them, so it was impossible to think this couldn't be resolved too.

On Saturday, 25 August we took Jade and Poppy, Melanie's horse, to an in-hand show. Poppy won the class for Best Manners for the young stock and third for conformation. Melanie, and her mother Dawn, were there too and were thrilled with this success, because Rebecca had been training Poppy for only three weeks. Poppy had been getting too pushy and Melanie hadn't been able to handle her. Melanie videoed Rebecca and Poppy.

It had occurred to me several times to buy a camera and video Rebecca in the paddocks with the horses, with her animals, painting and drawing, but I resisted the urge because it would have been an admission that we wouldn't have her in the world for much longer. Such a thought couldn't be allowed to take root. It is one of my enduring regrets now that I didn't do this. Apart from the video with Poppy, the only other one we have of Rebecca as a young adult is the one Sebastião took in Brazil. When Fabiano went back to Brazil after his first visit to Greendale, Rebecca and Natasha made a video of themselves singing, grooming the horses and generally clowning around. They were going to complete the video and send it to him, when Rebecca suddenly changed her mind. Four years later Natasha searched her father's garage for this video, but it was never found.

We were sitting in the sun watching Rebecca and Poppy, and chatting to Melanie and Dawn, when Mark and Susannah arrived. They stayed to watch some of the classes for a while then headed off to a winery to have a celebration lunch for Mark who'd just landed a new job.

When we went back home Rebecca and I took the horses for a two-hour trek along the river. It was perfect spring weather. Blue sky, warm sun and no wind. Rebecca showed me some banks on the river that I could ride up on Jade. I misunderstood and took him up what turned out to be the steepest bank of all. When I completed the manoeuvre without falling off Rebecca grinned at me. 'I'm so proud of you, Mum! I actually intended for you to ride up a *tiny* bank, not *that* one!'

We reached the gate of our paddocks as the sun was beginning to set and the sky turned pale gold. I thanked her for teaching me to ride.

'Without you, I'd never have had the opportunity to experience such a day as this,' I said.

Rebecca smiled. 'Will you continue riding when I'm not here?'

I shivered. 'Not here? You mean when you've left home?'

'Of course! Whaddya think I meant?'

'Just checking! But, the answer is probably no. Why?'

'You should,' she said. 'You're really good now.'

She went on to say that even when she did leave home she would need somewhere to keep her horses and we'd still ride together when she came back.

'One day I'll have my own stud and I'll need you to help me with it.'

I nodded.

# TEN

# A broken bowl

I picked Rebecca up from Art School and we set off home. She began weeping. I pulled in to the side of the road. She was getting frustrated, she said, because she could work only sporadically between chemo sessions. It was impossible for her to work that way. She needed to give her work 100 per cent otherwise it was too fragmented. She wanted to withdraw from study for the time being and concentrate on her recovery. She'd go back next year when all this was over. I said if that was what she wanted to do then it was fine by me.

At home she began spending her days working with her horses. Susannah asked her to paint a picture for her and bought the canvas and paints. Rebecca set it up on the easel and began. Bart also asked her to design a logo for the new electronics company he'd just started.

On Friday, 31 August we went to see the oncologist and got the results of the blood tests and CT scan. The CA 125 had decreased from 70 to 51 and the CEA from 45.5 to 34.1. While this was nowhere near as low as last month, the oncologist said it was nothing to worry about. The scan showed that two masses had slightly increased in size, but this may represent fluid rather than malignancy, he said.

We left feeling encouraged. At the beginning he hadn't been at all encouraging, saying this was a difficult tumour to treat and it wasn't usually responsive to chemo. Now he'd completely changed his attitude. He said he believed the treatment was effective and the fact that Rebecca looked well and was able to live a normal life was a very good prognostic factor. She'd begin another round of chemo the following week and he wanted to give her two more after that, and review the whole case in a couple of months. That would be when they'd decide whether or not to operate.

Our friend Helen, a nephrologist who'd lived in Texas for the last 20 years, suggested the tumour be reviewed at MD Anderson, one of the top cancer centres in Texas. I asked the oncologist about this and he said he'd arrange it, although it wouldn't change her treatment programme. The labs were now leaning to the idea of it being GI in origin, though they were still not certain.

Next day, 1 September, was the first day of spring. The darkness and bleakness of winter were retreating to be replaced by new life and energy. The landscape was still rain-saturated, but the grass was bright, and cherry and plum blossom were beginning to appear like loops of lace on the trees. The first green spears of daffodils, snowdrops and hyacinths were pointing above the earth. The days were lengthening. The birds were busy nest-building. We decided to redecorate the living room and ordered a new firebox to replace the old potbelly stove. I wanted to start gardening again, to clear away the dead leaves and plant a vegetable garden. I was starting to hope that by this time next year the cancer would have passed into the realm of nightmare.

Marilena wrote often. Two years after we left Brazil, Marilena married the man to whom she'd once been engaged when she was young. A chance meeting had rekindled their romance and they went to live in Maryland, in the USA. Marlí was now living in Marilena's house in Brazil and carrying on her reiki and massage business from there. Marlí told Marilena to let us know she was praying for Rebecca. Four months after leaving New Zealand Fabiano had met a girl, Roberta, a secretary at the language school where he'd taken his Cambridge Advanced English exams. Roberta sent Rebecca some crystals which had to be left in the light of the full moon and then dissolved in the bath. Rebecca laughed when she read the instructions, but thought it was sweet of Roberta to send them.

On 11 September, the day before my birthday, we went for a ride down to the river. When we returned, a thin slice of moon hung in the violet sky. The air was full of birdsong. Rebecca jumped off her horse and opened the gate.

'That was a great ride,' I said.

'The best,' she agreed.

She said she would unsaddle the horses, brush them and put away the gear if I'd run her a hot bath.

She stayed up late to finish an oil pastel drawing of Jade that she was doing for my birthday. I was reading in bed when she brought it in and showed me, smiling. 'D'ya like it?'

Jade's golden coat shone on the canvas and his eyes glinted with intelligence. I told her I loved it. This was the sixth oil pastel drawing she'd done of the horses and I suggested we go into town the next day to get them all framed. She grinned and went off to bed, happy.

Next morning Chris told me she was sitting on the side of her bed clutching her abdomen. She was in a lot of pain, so he would take her to hospital. I should just go to work and he'd let me know if it was anything serious. I went into her room. As usual, she was dismissive, but when pressed she said the pain had started soon after she'd gone to bed.

'Why didn't you tell me?'

'You need your sleep. You have to go to work.'

She shrugged off the pain and said it would wear off, only Dad was now insisting on going to the hospital. 'It's a lot of fuss about nothing!'

Later that morning I was leaving my classroom when I saw Chris walking up the street. One glance at his face sent my heart plummeting.

'Peritonitis,' he said.


Rebecca was lying on a bed waiting for the surgical team. She wasn't in pain now, she insisted.

The oncologist came into the room. 'Definitely peritonitis. Absolutely classic.'

He was a nice man. I just wished he hadn't looked so pleased when he said that.

A surgical registrar came in and examined Rebecca. As he left I asked if they were going to take out the tumours as well.

He blinked at me. 'Her abdomen is full of them. There's no point in taking out bits.' As he strode down the corridor in his blue overalls and white boots, he looked like an employee from the freezing works on his way to slaughter another sheep.

We sat in the waiting room for three hours while the operation was taking place, vaguely aware of people talking about twin towers in New York exploding. When it was over, the surgeon with whom Rebecca had wanted no further contact came in to tell us what had happened. They'd not only removed the burst appendix, he said, which they now realised had been the primary site of the cancer, the team had also taken out as much tumour as they could and washed Rebecca's abdominal cavity with the equivalent of bleach. He added that the surgeons were considering whether to do a temporary ileostomy to allow the bowel to heal.

'Temporary?'

He shrugged. 'Well, they're calling it temporary, but in my experience it's not always possible to reverse them.'

Always the Job's comforter, this one.

How long would Rebecca be in hospital?

A rare smile flickered across his face. 'Knowing her she'll be out tomorrow.'

We waited till she'd woken in HDU before we were allowed to see her. The nurse was trying to explain that she now had a bag attached to her stomach and what it was for. Rebecca was greatly interested in this and appeared to find the whole process fascinating. I couldn't believe her acceptance and apparent presence of mind.

Friends came to visit. A girl from the riding club brought horsey news. The sound of their laughter rang from the room. Art School friends were visibly shocked when they saw Rebecca's bald head and grey face. One girl went white, the other went red.

The doctors told us again this shouldn't have happened to Rebecca. They couldn't understand it. Appendix cancer was so rare that most doctors never saw a single case, not even in the more normal age group of 60+.

Carolyn Langlie-Lesnik's website on appendix cancer that I found seven years later stated that adenocarcinoma with signet ring cells was the rarest of the appendix cancers. The systemic chemotherapy used to treat it was the same used for colon cancer, but the disease was so rare no formal studies had been done on the efficacy of the chemotherapy. The appendix often ruptured early without patients being aware of it and the tumour spread quickly to other organs in the abdomen and peritoneum. Once cells became attached there they produced excessive amounts of a jellylike substance that eventually strangled other organs.

Although Carolyn had been given a poor prognosis she'd contacted the Memorial Sloan-Kettering Cancer Center in New York after reading about their successful new treatment. This involved removing all the tumours found in the abdomen along with affected organs while heated chemotherapy solution was directed into the abdomen during surgery. The doctor who performed her surgery had been part of a group that had published a study of this treatment, under the title *Surgical debulking and intraperitoneal chemotherapy for established peritoneal metastases from colon and appendix cancer*, in which the five year survival rate was shown to be 28 per cent. Carolyn felt this was a vast improvement on the zero odds she'd been given. After reaching her sixth year survival anniversary she set up a website in 2008 and wrote:

*There is no way I can return the favour to the many people who supported me. I
hope instead to 'pay it forward'. My creating this website is part of my attempt to
pay it forward to those newly diagnosed. My goal is to provide both information
and hope to those beginning this journey, the two things that were initially elusive
to me.*

After two weeks we took Rebecca home. She was cheerful and told us not to mention the word cancer any more. 'I just want to get out of this bloody dressing gown.'

The next morning she got up to have her breakfast. While I was in the shower I
heard the crash of broken pottery. I rushed into the kitchen to find Rebecca sitting on a
stool in tears. She'd flung her bowl across the room. It lay shattered on the floor.

She sobbed her despair and her anger at the surgeon who'd done the ileostomy. 'He
did it without *asking* me. I would have said *no.*'

'He saved your life.'

'I'd rather have *died.*'

In November, a month after the operation, Rebecca came out of her room covered in
paint and grinning from ear to ear. She'd started working on Susannah's painting a few
days before and had now completed it. It was a nude, painted in strong, vibrant colours.
The girl was standing with her back to the viewer. On the side of the painting were the
words: *She was here. Now is gone. All in all, life is cruel. Creation.* There were some other
indecipherable words and Rebecca wouldn't tell us what they were.

'None of it means anything,' she said. 'They're just words I made up.'

We drove over to Susannah's and Rebecca told her to wait outside till we'd hung the
picture. She was afraid Susannah wouldn't like it.

Susannah inhaled sharply. 'Oh, *Rebecca*! It's beautiful. It's exactly what I dreamt it
would be. You're so talented.'

Rebecca's face flushed with pleasure.

'So d'ya like it then?'

'Like it? I *love* it!' She took Rebecca into her arms and hugged her.

Mark and Susannah took her out to dinner to celebrate.

For the next two months she was well. She went up to Wellington to visit Benjamin for
a few days. He planned an itinerary for her which included most of the things he himself

found fascinating, such as walks through tunnels, a visit to see the underground cables of the cable car. She loved every minute. She especially loved that her brother had planned this so carefully. He was anxious that maybe he'd got it wrong and that she wouldn't be interested in the things he showed her. But she was, just because he'd done this for her.

As I listened to Benjamin on the phone describing where he'd taken Rebecca, I remembered the imaginary games they'd played as children. One of these games involved building and wiring a spaceship. We always knew they were immersed in this game when we saw them walking around in circles in the garden, lost in a world of their imagination. It went on for so many years that Susannah joked they'd still be playing the game when Benjamin went to university and had a girlfriend. The game didn't last that long, but when Dee appeared on the scene Rebecca resented her. 'She took my brother away,' she laughed when Benjamin and Dee got married, but by then she'd decided to like Dee. On what would have been Rebecca's 31st birthday, Benjamin had a plaque erected in the wildlife sanctuary in Wellington: *Rebecca Arnold, who loved everything in nature.* When he rang me to tell me this I wept. Wept because he'd had to do such a thing. And because he did do such a thing.

With a seven-year age gap Rebecca and Susannah never played together. 'She was like a doll I could dress up,' Susannah said. 'Then when she was a teenager I loved taking her shopping and getting her to try things on. I loved buying her things.' She regretted the times she'd seen Rebecca as an irritating younger sister who trailed after her and her best friend. 'But when she turned 20 I was starting to see her as an equal. A companion.'

Benjamin echoed this regret at sibling treatment seven years later, just before he flew to Sydney to start a new job. He remembered all the times he'd woken her in the middle of the night when they were children and got her to accompany him down the long spooky hall of our house and made her wait for him outside the bathroom. 'She stood there night after night in her bare feet on the cold lino,' he said. 'I wish I hadn't just got irritated and told her to go away.'

'Don't worry about it,' I said. 'If she were alive now, she'd think all that was highly amusing.'

A friend, Terri, came to visit with her son, Ben. They'd lived opposite us when we'd lived in town and Rebecca and Ben had gone to primary school together. When they were six Ben appeared at the front door with a bunch of flowers for Rebecca. They went to different high schools and on the rare occasions they met after that they didn't want to acknowledge each other's existence. When we bumped into them one day in town, just before we went to Brazil, both Rebecca and Ben sat red-faced and sullen while Terri and I chatted in a café. On the day they came to visit, Rebecca asked Ben if he'd like to go for a ride. I rode behind them with Terri and Chris walking. Ben hugged her before they left.

'They're like real adults now,' laughed Terri.

Rebecca suggested a picnic in Akaroa. On the way there she grew quiet and I sensed she was in pain, though she wouldn't admit it. As we started to get the picnic out she rubbed her stomach and said it was hurting a lot. We went to the clinic in Akaroa, but the GP was out on call and the nurse advised us to go to the hospital in Christchurch. By the time we completed the 90-minute trip back to town Rebecca was screaming. Chris drove frantically. Susannah and I could do nothing but repeat, 'We'll soon be there,' in a hideous echo of the phrase we'd used so many times on long holiday trips when they were children.

In ED a bowel blockage was diagnosed. This could be due to adhesions, or it could be the tumour spreading. The wait in ED, on this and many subsequent occasions, was interminable. When Rebecca was eventually admitted, she was taken to the cancer ward. It was full of white-faced elderly women in the latter stages of their disease. Rebecca blanched. I asked a nurse if there was a single room she could have instead. The nurse willingly found one, but I wondered why they'd thought it appropriate to put her in a ward with old ladies. Not for the startlingly insensitive reason the young house surgeon gave when he realised Rebecca was in a single room – 'This is better. You don't want to be in a room with smelly old people' – but because she didn't need to be reminded of the ravages cancer caused. The nurse apologised and explained that although there was a ward for children with cancer there was nothing appropriate for a young adult.

This trip marked the first of many. Each time we had to go through the same tedious bureaucratic procedure of waiting in a long queue while Rebecca rocked herself in agony as her details were entered on the computer. I asked if there was a way we could bypass this. No, there wasn't. On one such visit while we were waiting in a cubicle with Rebecca crying in pain, I asked the nurse to give her morphine. No, they couldn't, not until the doctor saw her. Well, when would that be? We had to be patient, she snapped, there were other sick people for the doctor to see; we weren't the only ones and they were after all checking Rebecca every half hour. I glanced at my watch. An hour had already passed between checks, but I was too tired to argue. I decided to file a complaint later. But I had no energy for that either.

In the weeks before Christmas, Rebecca was buoyed by the news Natasha was returning to New Zealand for a visit after two years in Australia. She was sitting in the sun by the swimming pool when Natasha arrived. As soon as Natasha saw her she wept, then apologised. 'It's just that I'm so happy to see you.' But to me she said, 'She's so thin!'

That evening they lay on the floor watching videos and eating sweets the way they had when they were teenagers. They planned to go back to Natasha's grandmother's house and 'pig out' doing the same there. However, the familiar pain started. Back to ED with Rebecca screaming in the car and Natasha, white-faced, holding her hand.

The site where the ileostomy bag was attached became red and itchy and sore. We visited the specialist nurse to see what could help. I expressed my concern at Rebecca's depression with this bag and the trouble it was giving her. Well, it was always the ones who refused to accept it that had the most trouble, she said tersely. Given her age, this was hardly surprising, I responded. She dismissed this. Oh no, she had other young girls who were very happy to wear a bag. It gave them quality of life.

We turned to more alternative practitioners. Someone recommended a couple who lived near us. They massaged her head and said she'd probably sleep after this treatment. She did, and vomited. They said that was a good sign. They recommended a man in Auckland, called Robert, who'd had remarkable cures with his machine that emitted light and high frequency sounds. I rang the number they gave me. The woman who answered was called Elaine. She sounded kind and told us when to come to Auckland. She also gave me the name of a woman near Christchurch who'd received this treatment. I could ring her if I liked. I did. This woman told us the session with Robert had helped her, but now she was ill again and was going back to his clinic in Auckland for more treatments. However, she'd bought herself a Rife machine which was similar to Robert's, and we were welcome to use it when she returned.

We travelled to Auckland. The naturopathic clinic run by Elaine and her husband, Alan, was the contact for the man who offered treatments with his machines. Robert was a genius, they said. They'd seen amazing cures in people the medical profession had given up on. Robert had built these machines himself and didn't even charge for their use. All that was needed was a small donation. They were kind and appeared genuine and organised some blood tests for Robert to diagnose.

Robert worked out of his small factory which produced herbal pills. He had three rooms, all equipped with different coloured lights in which music played constantly. This music consisted mostly of bird calls. Robert was in his sixties and had an abrupt, offhand manner. He warned Rebecca to stay out of hospital and to avoid chemotherapy treatment as this would cause more harm than good. Above all, she had to avoid morphine. Morphine would interfere with her body's ability to heal itself. He noticed she wore sunglasses. That was a mistake. The sun needed to get on the retina.

Over the following week I took Rebecca to Robert's clinic each morning. She sat in a room under a yellow light for two hours, listening to a combination of bird calls and music. Robert said he didn't work at the weekends so we'd just have to amuse ourselves. 'Go for walks on the beach,' he said. 'That will do you just as much good as sitting here.'

I asked him how much I should donate. Twenty dollars, he said. On the second visit I needed to clarify whether the 20 dollars was for each visit or a one-off donation. For each visit, of course, he laughed. Did I think I would be getting the other sessions free?

I expressed my doubts about him to Elaine. She assured me that was just his manner. He was brilliant, she said, and told me of all the cures she herself had witnessed. At her clinic she introduced us to an elderly Maori woman who offered to do spiritual healing.

I drove through Auckland trying to find the place with Rebecca reading the map and clutching her stomach in pain. She hadn't eaten all day and she'd stopped taking morphine, on Robert's advice. When we got out of the car she leaned against the bonnet and said she didn't think she could walk down the path. I helped her and we knocked at the door.

The room was already prepared with a massage table. A group of people stood around the table and laid their hands on her and prayed. The Maori woman said she often took a group around the cemeteries at night to heal tormented spirits. With a sinking feeling I wondered what on earth we were doing there. This woman said she wasn't impressed with Robert, which fuelled my own doubts even more. I wanted to go home. This was a waste of time. But what then? Who would help us, apart from Burje and Darina?

At the end of the hour-long session Rebecca sat up and said she felt great. She hopped off the table and said she was starving. My jaw dropped. Even the group seemed surprised. Rebecca ate sandwiches and drank tea. On the way back to our motel she was talkative and happy. I phoned home and said she was doing well. It seemed there had been a miracle that evening.

During the night she got up to be sick. She felt ill the next day and in the airport waiting for our plane back to Christchurch she was felled by a series of migraines. She sat on the floor looking skinny and washed out. In the plane she had another migraine. The flight attendant noticed and asked if he could help. I explained it was a migraine and he brought her oxygen. That cleared the migraine instantly. We were grateful for his kindness.

Chris was waiting for us in the arrival lounge. He told me later he hadn't recognised Rebecca at first because she looked so thin and ill. Just the migraine, I said. No, he said. More than that. Much more than that. Couldn't I see it? He was so shocked he went to see Peter, our GP, and asked for the truth. Peter told him she was dying. Rubbish! I said. That was defeatist talk. We must not communicate that to Rebecca. Miracles did happen. There was no reason why we couldn't beat this, but we needed to be committed.

I called the woman in Amberley with the Rife machine. Her daughter-in-law answered and told me she'd died while up in Auckland after visiting Robert's clinic. I rang Elaine who confirmed the woman had been very sick when she came to Robert. 'If only she'd made it through the weekend she might have been okay,' she said.

Elaine recommended a spiritual healer in Christchurch. I contacted her and she came out to spend time with Rebecca. Rebecca looked forward to these visits of Deidre and liked her enormously. Deidre stayed one weekend and gave her hands-on healing and crystals and peppered her conversation with talk about aliens with whom she was in contact. In the face of all evidence to the contrary I refused to doubt her. Chris's only comment was that at least Rebecca seemed to be getting some comfort out of it.

Burje saw Rebecca every day to give her acupuncture. We continued with the homeopathic remedies and the reiki. Not under any circumstances should we give her the calorie-rich health drinks suggested by the hospital, said Elaine. They were laden with all sorts of junk. She advised a juice-only diet for a couple of weeks so Rebecca could detox. But she was continuing to lose weight, I said. Not to worry, said Elaine. As soon as she could eat protein she would put the weight back on.

Rebecca hadn't painted for several weeks, but as Christmas approached she painted a horse for Elliot and wrote on it *A horse for Elliot*. We went to town for some red background paper and a frame. In the mall she said she wanted to buy a new keyring and chose one in the shape of a capital R with curls on each down stroke.

A few days after this we were sitting by the pool and she suddenly went indoors saying she felt like painting. After an hour or so I went in and saw her standing by her easel in the living room, painting with her hands. Her face was bright and streaked with paint. The painting showed the pale face of a young woman in profile. Behind her there was a swirling vortex of colour. It was as if the whole world had turned into wind. The painting disturbed me enormously, but Rebecca was pleased with it.

'I had no idea what I was going to paint. I don't know where that came from. I threw away my brush because I needed to get in there with my hands,' she beamed. 'It's for Burje.'

Another specialist was called in to review Rebecca's case. He told her the tumour was being tested again to see if it could be a more benign, slow-growing type of appendix cancer called pseudomyxoma peritonei. If that were the case, he said, the outlook was far more positive. That type of cancer was treatable. He'd been treating a patient with that condition for 20 years. 'She's dying now, of course,' he added casually to Rebecca. 'She's in a ward here at the moment.'

Once again I swallowed down my indignation that a doctor could drop in that information so carelessly.

When the results came through, the team of doctors who were caring for Rebecca scheduled a meeting with her. She didn't want to go to the meeting and asked Chris and me to go instead. To authorise this she had to write a letter. When we all assembled, one of the doctors frowned and asked where Rebecca was. Another doctor showed him the letter. He frowned again and muttered that this was most irregular. He then went on to tell us that the results had shown that the cancer was unfortunately not pseudomyxoma peritonei. The disease had progressed and was now filling Rebecca's abdominal cavity. There was no point in performing further surgery. She had only a few months left. He was very sorry. What about more chemo? I asked. He shrugged. No, chemo simply knocked off a few cells. Rebecca's oncologist sat with his head slumped on his chest. When he raised it he had tears in his eyes. He said he'd like to try a course of another chemotherapy, irinotecan. That would give her more time.

How much more?

About two months.

The surgeon said he'd schedule an operation after the New Year to try to reverse the ileostomy. He warned us it might not be possible, but he would do his best.

We gave Rebecca an edited version of the meeting and told her about the irinotecan. She was adamant she wanted no more chemotherapy and would use alternative therapies instead. When we told the oncologist he arranged for a palliative care doctor to see her.

Kate, as this doctor told us to call her, was young, cheerful and positive. Palliative care was not about the beginning of the end, she said, it was about providing the best quality of life possible. She advised Rebecca that she could wear a Fentanyl patch on her arm. This was an opioid that would provide continuous pain relief. It was not funded by Pharmac, so we would have to pay for it ourselves if we wanted it. Yes, we did want it. Rebecca asked if she'd still be able to go swimming with the patch on her arm. Kate looked surprised and said she'd have to check.

'No one's ever asked me about swimming before,' she said. 'Most of my patients are elderly and they don't care about swimming!'

Rebecca laughed with her.

When we went back to the hospital next day the nurse told us Rebecca had woken in the night screaming. She'd been trying to get out of bed and had sent the IV stand crashing to the floor. When I asked Rebecca about it she said she'd woken up in pitch blackness. She didn't know where she was or even who she was.

'Why didn't you get the nurse to phone me? We would've come straight in,' I said.

'I thought about it and I wanted to, but it was two in the morning. You need your sleep.'

I made her promise that if such a thing ever occurred again she would ring me immediately.

She promised.

'Did you think you were dying?' I asked.

'I thought I already had.'


Benjamin, Dee and Elliot came to stay with us for Christmas, and Benjamin and Rebecca decorated the Christmas tree. On Christmas Day, Susannah and Mark came over. Rebecca was disturbed by Elliot's crying so she stayed in bed. She got up later to eat some ham, though Elaine had given her a strict diet of no protein. We had bought a special juicer so we could juice carrots and beetroot and fruit. Robert had said ordinary juicers were useless. It had to be this particular brand. Rebecca said frequently while following this diet, 'I could *kill* for a bacon sandwich.'

After dinner she put her bikini on, not caring about the top of the bag being visible and went for a swim.

On New Year's Eve, Grant and his girlfriend, Kirsten, and Bart came out to Green-dale. We wrapped Rebecca up in blankets and they all stayed out by the pool to see the New Year in. Grant and Bart clowned around in the water and the garden was once again filled with the sound of laughter.

In January Chris and I took Rebecca to Auckland again so she could have more treatment with Robert. At our motel we met a middle-aged woman called May who'd travelled there from Australia with her elderly mother-in-law. May had bowel cancer. Robert had been strongly recommended to them by a friend in Australia, they said. We'd hired a car so we gave them lifts to the clinic. May said she'd been married only a few months before.

'It was a lovely wedding,' she said wistfully.

The treatment didn't seem to be helping, she complained, and her pain was increasing.

Robert repeated to Rebecca that morphine would make her worse and she must make an effort to stop using it again and at all costs keep away from hospitals. She took off the Fentanyl patch.

She wanted to go to Kelly Tarlton's Underwater World and the zoo. At the zoo we had to get a wheelchair for her as the effort of walking was too much. However, next day she walked for two kilometres on the beach and bathed in the sea. For several weeks Chris had been reading to her at night from *Lord of the Rings*, one of her favourite books as a child. She said the sound of his voice took her deep into the story until she forgot about her pain. Now he told me he was coming to the end of the story and he was dreading it.

'Why?' I asked.

'They die.'

Rebecca woke up one night crying in pain so we went to the ED, which fortunately we'd made a point of locating on our arrival. There we met nurses and doctors who, for some unaccountable reason, seemed kinder and more thoughtful than some of those we'd experienced in Christchurch. As the nurse X-rayed Rebecca she said, 'Poor thing, her spine's showing.' The surgeon said he'd operate to clear the adhesions and at the same time reverse the ileostomy, but first we had to wait for the result of the scan.

The registrar showed us into a room and asked us to sit down. I knew by the expression on his face and the tone of his voice that the operation wouldn't take place. When the consultant came in he said he couldn't operate because the tumour had spread too far.

'Go home,' he said softly to Rebecca. 'Go back to your family and friends.'

She cried. Chris and I sat barely breathing.

When we returned to Christchurch, May phoned from Auckland to say she too had had to go to ED and they'd dosed her up with enough morphine to enable her to make the journey home to Australia. 'I have six weeks left,' she said.

I didn't tell Rebecca.

# ELEVEN

# Wild ducks and bonfires

The ileostomy reversal was scheduled for 13 February. The surgeons warned Rebecca it might not be possible to achieve, but they were prepared to do all they could. I emailed Robert about this. He responded that the doctor's advice was a warning and Rebecca should proceed cautiously at this stage. Indications were that the bowel would function if the operation did go ahead, but he advised delay while she was in a healing mode. The lymphocytic pockets in the colon were not cancer, he said, and there was no tumour in that region. Rather, the obstacles intimated were physical ones for the surgeons. Her ovary was normalising in function and would be fully functional by Easter, although surgical trauma could delay this.

On 5 February I emailed him again:

*Rebecca has decided to go ahead with the operation which is scheduled for*
*Wednesday, 13th Feb. She said she had thought it over very carefully after*
*listening to everyone's opinions and still remains convinced that she will not*
*recover until the bag is removed and the ileostomy closed and that it has to*
*happen sooner rather than later. The palliative care doctor rang me yesterday to*
*express her anxiety about the operation. She has not yet seen the CT scans which*
*the North Shore Hospital was supposed to send down last week, but didn't. She*
*commented that even if there was a slight reduction in the size of the tumour mass*
*in Rebecca's abdomen she would feel more optimistic. I told her that we believed*
*the cancer was not active and that the tumours were gradually being re-absorbed.*

*She commented that she was very surprised that Rebecca was still looking well almost three months after the doctors who reviewed her case declared that she had a very aggressive tumour and had only a few months left. She said, 'I don't understand how this holistic care you're getting from Auckland is working, but it most definitely is and I hope that all the doctors here are proved wrong and the Auckland clinic is right.'*

*A spiritual healer called Deidre (recommended by Elaine) has been working with Rebecca since November. When she saw her last Friday she said she suspected that the abdominal mass that the Auckland doctors had seen on the scan might be a tapeworm. What do you think?*

Robert responded briefly that there was no cancer, and no tapeworms. Her ovary function had now normalised, he said, and wished her good luck for the operation, which he was sure would be successful.

Deidre's son rang to say his mother was dancing naked on the lawn and he was about to ring a psychiatrist. He rang later that night to say she'd been taken to the mental hospital and could we please drop off the crystals she'd left with us. Rebecca was devastated. We explained that Deidre was manic-depressive. Now we knew she was mentally ill we could only feel compassion. Chris wrapped his arms around both of us, both physically and figuratively. It is a measure of this lovely man that he never once said *I told you so*, not even when I sent away for Noni juice that was claimed to have miraculous cancer-curing properties.

The day before Rebecca's operation my friend Marj wrote from England:

*Needless to say I had been wondering how things were and had intended to contact you this week. I must tell you about something that happened last night not long before you sent the e-mail. I was watching Songs of Praise on the television and during the singing of one of the hymns there was a particular point when a very strong image came into my mind of me standing over Rebecca with my hands on her head and my hands felt really hot. There was also another point when someone was being interviewed. She had been in hospital with her very sick baby and had been told to go and pray in the hospital chapel if she had any faith. She went and instead of praying for the baby to recover she asked for strength to cope with whatever the outcome was. These two things really stuck in my mind and I had them on my mind all night. I don't know exactly what they meant but I do pray that you will all have strength to face whatever is to come. Wednesday is Bethan's birthday and she promised me that she would start the day with a prayer for Rebecca as of course we all will. I've also contacted the healing group at church and they will too. Rebecca must be a very brave and special person and we send her and you lots of love.*

Chris and I waited in a small room off the operating theatre. After three hours we saw the registrar walking past. We ran out and asked him how things had gone. In the corridor he explained he was very sorry, but the surgeon hadn't been able to reverse the ileostomy. The colon was full of cancer. It was just like tissue paper. I wanted to scream, but there was a side room full of people all listening to the conversation.

Rebecca opened her eyes in the recovery room. She smiled when she saw us. 'When are they going to operate?'

'Darling, they couldn't do it.'

She frowned. 'Why have they postponed it?'

'They haven't postponed it. It's not possible at this time to do it. They cancelled the operation.'

She stared at me then lifted the sheet and felt her stomach. She frowned and turned her face away from us. I glanced at Chris. His face was grey and tired. We leaned into each other and touched Rebecca's arm. Her skin shivered as if we'd burned her.

In the ward she refused to speak to anyone. When the surgeon came in she wouldn't look at him. He kept saying how sorry he was. I talked to Kate and cried and cried. She told me I needed to tell Rebecca she was dying.

I sat on the side of her bed and started telling her that I wanted her to live more than anything, but that if she wanted to let go she could and I wouldn't cling to her. If she wanted to fight we would be right there for her. I just wanted to let her know that whatever she decided was right for her was okay with us.

She sat up then and said forcefully, 'I'm not dying *yet* you know!' and went on to tell me this kind of comment did not help her or me and she didn't want people to talk as if she were dying. Unfortunately, the surgeon walked in right then and she immediately closed her eyes and wouldn't talk to him. As soon as he left Kate came in and got the same response. Then in came one of my friends who'd just heard the news from Chris and had rushed to the hospital. She came in crying and when Rebecca saw her she closed her eyes and pretended she'd gone to sleep. I took the friend for a coffee because Rebecca was overloaded dealing with other people's reactions.

Next day we took her home. She was silent on the journey back. She watched a video, still very silent, then went to bed and slept for five hours. Susannah and Mark came for dinner and Rebecca got up at 7.30, greeted them cheerfully, sat at the table and had dinner with us and chatted and laughed. When they left she walked to the front door to say goodbye and then watched another video with me, laughing at the comedy and eating a snack of cheese and crackers. Chris and I just shook our heads at each other.

The following morning Chris went outside to chop wood. Rebecca appeared with a couple of pillows, paper and a pencil. She lay down in the garden near Chris, scribbling on her paper. I asked if she was comfortable there and she answered cheerfully that she'd decided to be positive and get on with her life. She liked being near her father for company, she said, and she was writing a list of all the things she wanted to do. At the top of the list she'd written 'A best friend necklace for Natasha'. Next, she'd compile a photo album of all the horses she'd ever owned. She'd label the album Beija-Flor.

'Beija-Flor?'

'I'm Beija-Flor, right? It's what I was going to call my horse stud.'

Once again I could hardly keep pace with the changes in her mood. She spent several hours on the computer designing name labels for each horse, and each page was decorated with little borders of prancing horses. She also worked on another stylised design for a horse on the computer. Friends came to visit and she talked and laughed with them. She said she hated the way people talked to her in the hospital, all the tears and hand-wringing, and didn't want that. She started drinking high energy food supplements and put on five kilograms in a week.

After a few days she was subdued again. Chris told me she'd said there were some new lumps on her abdomen and made him promise not to tell me. She also told Sue, our neighbour, about these lumps and Sue suggested they went on a horse ride down to the river. That was her last ride. She said the level of pain was increasing and she'd been taking more morphine.

On February 16 and 17, Rebecca asked me to sleep in the garden with her, under the stars. We brought out sleeping bags and quilts and hot water bottles and dozed in the sun loungers until night fell, occasionally talking. Before falling asleep she told me her favourite sounds were the wind in the trees and the spikers, the young deer, calling in the autumn evenings. We listened to them now as we drifted off to sleep. She woke me once in the night.

'Mum, look up.'

I looked up at the sky, crammed with stars.

'Isn't it beautiful?' she whispered.

'So very beautiful,' I said.

'Do you remember when we went to Disneyland, on the way to Brazil? On one of those rides we went on? All the stars?'

Yes, I did remember. She'd said the same thing then: 'Mum! Look up!'

But that was a world away; when she had the whole world to look forward to and a lifetime to live.

The next evening we took Rebecca over the road in the wheelchair the hospital had lent us, to have a few drinks with Sue and her husband, John. They lit a bonfire. We sat by the bonfire listening to music, watching flights of wild ducks in the sky, a silver slice of moon and the first pale stars. In the warmth and crackling of the fire it was easy to feel everything was normal. John set off some firecrackers and in the illuminated red flare Rebecca's face was relaxed and happy.

David wrote to Rebecca from Brazil:

*Today I took two children up to the little library that we have upstairs in the Academy. When kids have to wait for their turn to ride, or when they are afraid of horses we often take them there. There are books and magazines about horses and they always enjoy their visit there. Today the little girl that was with me noticed the horse picture on the wall that you painted. It is so colorful and bright and she thought it was beautiful. I think it changed her attitude and made her more interested in riding and increasing her contact with horses. I thought that would make you happy since horses are so important to you too. Thank you again so much for the picture and the positive effects that it has on the youngsters that come to ride with us.*

One night we were woken up by the sound of laughter. We got up and found Rebecca sitting on the floor in the hall. She was laughing and talking, though her speech had been slurred and faint all day. She said she didn't know whether she was dreaming or not, or whether she was looking at her past, present or future, or if she was even dreaming the words she was saying to me right now. She thought she'd been somewhere, but she couldn't remember where. She said she wished she could remember because it had been lovely there.

Fabiano wrote to say he was coming to New Zealand to stay with us for a month. I wrote back to say how happy Rebecca was with that news and warned him of what he would see.

*Only a short time ago the house was filled with her laughter and personality. Now she can scarcely smile. I'm sorry to be so sad, but you need to be prepared for what you will see here. Just be your natural self with Rebecca and she will feel at ease with you.*

He left his job and his girlfriend and arrived on 1 March. Chris picked him up at the airport and when he entered the house he was smiling and happy to be back. He asked where Rebecca was and could he please see her? When I told Rebecca he'd arrived, her face lit up. When he saw her he hugged her and asked how she was feeling.

'Oh, I've been better,' she said airily.

I left them.

When he came out his face was grey. He hadn't realised, he said, that she was so ill. Not like this. Not so thin. Not so sick.

The district nurse arrived to give the morphine injection.

Fabiano sat with his head in his hands.

Over the next week we had barbecues in the garden with Rebecca wrapped up in quilts on the sun lounger. John and Sue set up loudspeakers so we could play CDs. Fabiano baked *pão de caixo*, a Brazilian cheesebread. Rebecca said, 'I've been hanging out for these,' and wolfed several of them down. Chris lit sparklers.

On other days we took her over to John's in a wheelchair and sat in his garden in front of a brazier. Rebecca loved those times of talk and music and laughter. But on one of those days we'd just arrived at John's when she said she wanted to return home as she was in pain. Chris wheeled her as quickly as he could across the road. Fabiano and I hurried behind. Before Chris got her to the house we heard her wail. Fabiano, who hadn't heard this before, sucked in his breath at the sound.

I asked her if she'd like to sleep with me that night and she said she would. I lay awake next to her thinking of how she'd loved lying in bed with me when she was a child. Back in the days when I believed I had the power to keep her safe. But there was no sticking plaster big enough to mend her now, no hug wide enough to protect her. *Eat all your vegetables and you'll grow up big and strong. Don't talk to strangers. Come home before midnight. Don't drive too fast. Don't gallop bareback. Wear a helmet when you play ice hockey. Wear sun screen or you'll have skin like leather by the time you're thirty.* But this enemy? There wasn't a thing we could do to stop it destroying her. And not a thing all the doctors and all the alternative practitioners in the world could do. And this knowledge crushed me.

She was restless and woke frequently and started to get out of bed.

'Where are you going?' I asked.

'I'm disturbing you too much,' she said. 'You need your sleep.'

I asked her where she'd prefer to be, in her own room or with me.

'With you. I'm scared I might die in the night.'

'I'm right here. You're safe,' I lied.

In the morning as she got out of bed I saw her left leg had a blue tinge. I called the GP from Darfield. He thought it might be a blood clot and called the ambulance to take her straight to ED.

Again the interminable wait. The forms to fill in. By the time we saw a doctor Rebecca was crying in pain. She couldn't bear anyone to touch her leg. Fabiano stood at the end of the bed fighting back tears. He'd seen that one of the doctors he'd been friends with during his three month internship at the hospital was on duty that night, so left a message for him. This doctor now appeared in the cubicle. It was the same registrar who'd given us the news that the surgeon hadn't been able to reverse the ileostomy. When he realised that Rebecca was the girl Fabiano had talked so much about two years ago he reeled in shock.


A registrar came in to tell Rebecca that the X-ray had revealed a massive blood clot in her leg which extended right across her abdomen under her heart. He told her there wasn't much point in giving her Heparin to thin the blood as this could cause the tumours to bleed.

'Basically, you take your pick,' he said airily. 'The cancer or the blood clot.' And he left.

Rebecca looked at me and wept. 'There's no *point* in me making plans for the future. There *isn't* any.'

I found the doctor and berated him furiously for his choice of words and his lack of sensitivity. Tears sprang to his eyes. He apologised. Another doctor bustled in with a form and, barely out of Rebecca's earshot, told us he assumed we wouldn't want her resuscitated in the event she had a heart attack. Next came the consultant who told us she had kidney failure and wouldn't survive more than a couple of days.

Rebecca was admitted to the ward and she was given heparin injections to thin her blood. The swelling in her leg gradually decreased and the colour returned to normal. Her kidney function improved and she began to eat and drink. Fabiano never left her bedside. He massaged her feet and brought DVDs for her to watch on his laptop. One of her horsey friends came to visit and Rebecca sat up talking and laughing with her. She commented, along with the nurses, that Rebecca's boyfriend was very handsome.

'He's not my boyfriend,' Rebecca laughed.

'But you look so close. We assumed he must be your brother or your boyfriend.'

Grant and Bart came every day. Natasha had by now arrived back in New Zealand having made the decision to leave Australia for good as soon as she'd heard that Rebecca was deteriorating. With all the laughter that filled the hospital room it was hard to imagine the dramas of the last week.

Rebecca asked Susannah to find a necklace in the form of a heart on which was engraved 'Best Friends'. This heart could be separated and each half worn on a silver chain. When Natasha visited her in hospital, Rebecca gave her one of the hearts. Natasha couldn't keep back her tears. They each fastened their silver chains around their necks.

We took Rebecca in the wheelchair along the Avon River which ran by the hospital. It was the same path we'd walked on with her and Bruno five years before, the day we'd gone to see *Titanic*. Then, she'd worn a mauve miniskirt and black halter top and riding boots. Her blonde hair had cascaded around her shoulders and she'd walked in long strides laughing at a joke Bruno was telling.

Susannah had nudged me. 'Those men keep staring at Rebecca!'

'Well, she's nineteen.'

'But she's my baby sister. I feel like punching them!'

We'd all laughed.

We stopped now to look at the ducks in the river. Passers-by glanced at Rebecca's bald head and skeletal figure and quickly looked away. One whispered, 'It's nice that they let them out, isn't it?'

Them?

Nice?

After five days of being rehydrated Rebecca gained five kilograms and we could take her home. As soon as we got her home she felt very ill and we got up with her several times during the night. The next day she wanted to go back to hospital again. The main problem was acute pain. It was time for a morphine pump to be attached to her arm which would administer morphine over 24 hours. The district nurses would come daily and they'd show us how to give extra morphine by injection if she needed it.

The following morning we arrived at the hospital to find Rebecca sitting up in bed watching a nature documentary and drinking a cup of tea.

'I ate a whole bowl of porridge,' she told me cheerfully.

She became very dozy after that and slept most of the day as a result of the increased morphine and sleeping pills. When she woke up she vomited. The weight she'd gained was rapidly disappearing so she was given anti-emetics. The doctors told us it was possible her intestines were too obstructed to function now.

Fabiano's mother arranged for 'spiritual surgery' with her Spiritist Church in Brazil with a follow up on the next three Fridays. We contacted all our friends around the world and asked them to pray for Rebecca on that day.

The 'spiritual surgery' took place from 12.00 to 2.00pm on Friday, 15 March. Chris sat outside the door to prevent interruptions and Fabiano prayed in Portuguese as I read some passages from the *Book of Spirits*, in English. The atmosphere was very calm and peaceful. Afterwards Rebecca said she was hungry and sent Chris out for a pizza. She said she'd felt calm and positive during the proceedings. She was talkative, happy and lively for the rest of the day and evening, and eating and drinking ravenously. We weighed her and found she'd regained the five kilos.

Chris brought her home next day, but the journey in the car was very uncomfortable, exacerbated by a half-hour wait at the pharmacy. The chemist read the prescription and told Chris that if he ever needed any medication rapidly all he had to do was ask. He'd be more than willing to open up the pharmacy if we needed immediate access, he said.

By the time they got home Rebecca was in a lot of pain. She was awake and in pain most of the night and the next day asked to go back to the hospital. We took her back and once again she started to pick up by evening. Next day she was lethargic, sleepy, not eating, and drinking only a little and requesting morphine every hour or two. In the evening she had a migraine and was sick, but after the nurse gave her some oxygen she felt better and started to talk and laugh. One of the nurses brought in a little white puppy for her to see.

'Against regulations,' she said, 'but what the hell!'

It cheered Rebecca up enormously. She loved the dog and said she would like one like that for her birthday the following month.

She told me she was sorry for spoiling Fabiano's holiday.

'It can't have been much fun for him stuck in hospital with me all the time.'

'You're the only reason he come back.'

She considered this in silence.

'You know, Mum, I was really horrible to him when he was here two years ago.'

'He understands all that.'

'I see tears in his eyes every day.'

I nodded.

'You know … if I was well, I would have him now.'

I raised an eyebrow.

'I never realised what he was really like before.'

He was special, I agreed. She asked me if I'd tell him what she felt. I suggested she do so herself.

She shook her head. 'It wouldn't be fair on him. I'm not well.'

'He might still like to know.'

She asked me to send him in.

When he came back out of the room his face was wet, but he was smiling.

# TWELVE

# No more miracles

Rebecca was now only 50 kilograms. Her eyes were like pale blue milk, her face pallid, and her limbs like something out of Belsen. The only part of her that looked substantial was the huge mass of tumour extending her abdomen. She told the nurse she wanted to be rehydrated.

I wrote to Robert on 26 March to ask his opinion. Robert didn't reply to me directly, but forwarded his response to Alan at the clinic, who wrote that the key ingredient was what Rebecca wanted to do. Their opinion was that it was never too late for a recovery, but even if she did not, then we would have the benefit of knowing that we'd done all we humanly could.

The nurse rang the doctor at Darfield who came out to attach the IV drip. After 300ml went in, the drip blocked. The nurse was going to put saline through it to flush it, but at that point Rebecca decided she didn't want the drip in and she would try to continue with drinking by mouth. I urged her to eat. She shook her head. 'Believe me, Mum, it's not that I don't want to. I'm hungry all the time. I'm thirsty all the time. But I can't.'

Fabiano's mother, Cleuza, had organised follow-up spiritual surgery. While Fabiano read the prayer Rebecca lay in bed with her eyes closed. Afterwards she said she had the strong impression that Cleuza was in the room with her at that moment. Fabiano emailed his mother to tell her this and she reported that she had indeed been praying for Rebecca at that precise moment and the fact Rebecca could sense it was a very good indicator of the success of the 'surgery', on a spiritual level.

Benjamin, Dee and Elliot arrived and stayed in John's guesthouse over the road from us. At night Rebecca was often more comfortable sleeping in the La-Z-Boy chair in the living room. Chris stayed up at nights with her and Benjamin and Fabiano took turns with this so Chris could get some sleep. Rebecca often dozed during the day, but at nights she was wakeful and restless. Though I was exhausted I was terrified to sleep in case she should die when I wasn't near her.

Bart and Grant and Natasha visited and took Rebecca over to John's garden in the wheelchair. She smiled and joked with them, pumping her hand, saying, 'Parp, parp,' when she wanted them to turn left or right. Grant told me the thing he missed most was hearing her bubbly laugh. In the privacy of Rebecca's room they said what they needed to.

They brought some balloons that could be blown into animal shapes. Rebecca was delighted and tried to blow one herself. She couldn't manage to get enough air into her balloon and said, in tears of frustration, 'I can't even blow up a balloon animal.' The boys felt terrible that their great idea had caused her more distress. Mark took the balloon she'd been blowing and found it was faulty. He demonstrated that he couldn't get it to inflate either. That made Rebecca feel a little better, but she was worn out and went to her room to lie down. When I went in later she said, 'I'm so scared. I think I might die any day.'

I asked her why she thought that.

'Why else are they hanging around? It's like they're waiting for me to cark it!'

'No. They're here because they love you,' I said.

She nodded. 'Well, I have no intention of carking it. I have too much stuff to do.'

When Bart visited another day they stayed in the garden laughing and chatting. However, Rebecca had sudden pain that necessitated another call to the ambulance, another visit to ED, another interminable wait with her crying in pain at yet another bowel obstruction.

Back at home she slowly, inexorably wasted away. Yet still she talked about the future, and all the horse training she planned on doing when she was better. As I helped her out of the bath one evening she caught sight of her reflection in the mirror. Her enormous eyes in a pale skeletal face.

'Oh my *God*!' she said. 'I look *horrible*! I don't look like *me* anymore!' The effort of getting her back to bed exhausted her, so that was the last of the baths. I washed her in bed after that. Some days she could speak only in slurred whispers. She said, 'I can't swallow and I can't talk. Why?'

'You're so weak now. If only you could try to eat a little.'

'I wish I could.'

One day she said, 'Something has changed. Something else is going on. I think I might die any day and I don't want to die.'

Hearing this broke my heart.

Melanie brought over the video she'd taken of Rebecca and Poppy winning the Best Manners class. Another time she brought her new kittens over. Rebecca drifted off to sleep stroking the kittens on her lap.

John brought some fireworks and flares over to set off one evening and we wheeled Rebecca out onto the verandah to watch. We hadn't realised they'd explode with such a bang and Chris, who'd been trying to snatch some much-needed sleep after staying up with Rebecca all night, came storming out demanding to know what the hell we were playing at. Despite our contrition we couldn't help laughing at his red, annoyed face. Rebecca was particularly contrite, but when Chris went back to bed she doubled over with laughter, at the same time saying how guilty she felt about doing this. We didn't care. To see her laugh like that was worth any discomfort.

In the days before Fabiano's departure she asked us to take her out to see the horses. Red reached over the gate to sniff at her in the wheelchair. Despite her weakened state she raised her hand to remind him of his manners and to warn him not to invade her personal space. When he took a step back she reached out and stroked his nose, murmuring to him softly. Bug leaned his big head over the gate and she blew gently into his nostrils. Fabiano wheeled her over to John's paddock to see Kit and Jade. She hadn't seen Kit for several weeks and marvelled at how much she'd grown, how thick and beautiful her mane was. She laughed to see how protective Jade was of Kit. Satisfied that all the horses were looking well, she was happy to return home.

I could no longer bear to go shopping and see crowds of healthy young people striding about, calling to each other in that loud, careless way they have. We inhabited a different world now. The phone didn't ring as often and when it did, the voice on the other end was hushed and afraid to ask how things were going. Rebecca spent most of her time in the living room, so it was difficult to answer inquiries about her. On the odd occasion I took the phone into another room she looked at me suspiciously.

The autumn weather continued warm and golden. As the leaves turned red and dropped from the trees my heart was so heavy I had to go out into the paddocks to cry where Rebecca couldn't see me. One day as I was standing there, stroking the horse, a couple of neighbours passed by and stopped to talk. They chatted about their holiday and where they might go next. I tried to feign interest, but it was a reminder of how much my world had shrunk. Just a few months later, one of these neighbours was killed in a road accident.

Fabiano had to leave to go to his new job. On Monday, 1 April, Rebecca insisted on going with us to the airport to see him off. We all stood outside the car not looking at each other as he and Rebecca said their goodbyes. We went into the airport with him while Benjamin stayed with Rebecca.

'The last time you waved goodbye to me here, I was very sad because she didn't want me,' he wept. 'But I promised her I would come back one day and wait for her. And now … only two years later … this?'

But we could offer no comfort.

Back home Rebecca said she wished he hadn't gone. We missed him too, not least because he had alternated on the night shifts with Chris. Now Benjamin stayed up all night with her, emptying the commode the hospital had given us, whenever necessary. He, the most squeamish of all our children, did this without turning a hair. They talked about films, their childhood, songs they liked, Benjamin's future plans.

She said she was sick of being this way. 'It's gone on too long. I just want it to go one way or the other. This is not me any more. I don't even look like me. I've had enough.'

I held her hand and said I wished I could take this from her. That I wished it had happened to me and not her. She looked shocked. 'Well, I don't!' she said.

I asked if she wanted to give up now or continue fighting. She thought for a minute and said, 'I'll continue fighting.'

The doctors told me that it was time to stop fighting. 'Let nature take its course,' they said. They kept urging me to tell her that death was approaching. I responded that if she asked me that question I'd answer honestly, but unless she asked I wouldn't bring up the subject. Around this time I heard an interview on the radio where a mother said the doctors had told her to tell her nine-year-old son he was dying. Children and young people had a very pragmatic view about death, they said and always knew when they were dying. The mother, against her better judgement, told her child the truth. The frightened boy asked what dying would be like and she told him it was just like falling asleep. For the six months before he died he was too frightened to close his eyes. She regretted now not listening to herself.

Listening to oneself was the key, I thought. For me, it felt right to wait until Rebecca let me know she was ready to have this conversation. How could I otherwise introduce the subject of her dying when I didn't even believe it myself?

On Tuesday, the day after Fabiano left, she asked to go to Darfield Hospital to be rehydrated. That had always worked in the past months when she was feeling weak and tired. Susannah came to say goodbye to her there. 'I've made a chocolate cake,' she said. 'It's in the kitchen. When you go home you can have a piece.' Rebecca smiled and said she was looking forward to it.

On Thursday she said she wanted to go on a picnic to a place we'd once visited on the way to Geraldine, where she'd thrown chunks of ice into the frozen lake. 'I want to get out of this bloody nightie and put some proper clothes on,' she said.

Her tracksuit hung off her emaciated body as if from a wire coat hanger.

I suggested Whitecliffs instead. It was only half an hour away and we'd spent many happy days picnicking there when she was a child.

We'd arrived in New Zealand in 1976 with Benjamin aged two, and Susannah six. A few months after settling in Christchurch, we thought about having another baby. One day we went to Whitecliffs for a picnic with another English family we'd met. They had a little daughter and a new baby girl. The beautiful river setting, the space, the peace and quiet of the day, the warm smell of the new baby, convinced me New Zealand would be a good place to raise three children.

During my pregnancy I didn't know whether I was carrying a boy or a girl. Rebecca was the only name I wanted and I had no idea what I'd call the baby if it were a boy. The week before I went into labour I kept seeing the letter R everywhere I looked, and I became convinced the baby would be a girl. She was born with her eyes wide open and, true to the character she would become, no crying.

'Hello Rebecca,' I said to the crumpled red face.

The cleaners who came in saw me gazing at her asked if she was my first.

'No, my third.'

'Yer third? Yer look like she's yer first, eh?'

When my children were small, they liked to ask me, 'How much do you love us?'

'Oh. As high as the sky. As deep as the ocean. As wide as the world.'

'Will you always love us? Even when we're bigger than you?'

'Always and forever.'

As we packed the morphine with the picnic, Rebecca said with a big grin, 'No more health food. I want white bread and a bag of chips and lemonade.'

At Whitecliffs we helped her outside to sit in the wheelchair. I prepared her sandwich. She couldn't eat it. She couldn't swallow the lemonade. She asked to go back home.

'I'm so sorry,' she said.

'For what?'

'For ruining your day out.'

In the middle of my protestations she thanked us for everything we'd done for her. She'd been a pain, she said, but we'd been so kind to her and so patient and she really appreciated it. I would have scooped her up in my arms then if I hadn't been afraid of snapping her in two.

'If you've been grumpy at times, you've had every right to be,' I said. 'Nobody minds. We wanted to take this from you, but we can't. All we can do is love you. And it doesn't feel enough.'

'It *is* enough,' she said.

Back home she sat by the pool in the sun with Chris. I was about to go out and join them when the phone rang. It was Sebastião from Brazil. His voice was anxious. I put the phone down after a few minutes, but Rebecca had already come back indoors. The light was too bright, she said and she went to bed.

On Friday a friend arrived with a bunch of flowers. When he saw Rebecca he asked her how she was.

'I've been better,' she grinned and thanked him for the beautiful flowers.

As I said goodbye to him on the porch I cried and he was close to tears himself. 'At least you've got two other children,' he said. 'If this was me – well, I've only got one.'

He meant well, so I said nothing.

Back in the house I went to help Rebecca on the commode and she fell back on the bed, her eyes rolling upward. I called out to Benjamin, but by the time he rushed into the room she'd regained consciousness.

Later that evening she had a sudden pain in her chest. While we were waiting for the nurse to come out she whimpered, 'Help me, please help me.' I called the doctor. He thought it might be a blood clot in her heart, but the medication the nurse gave her settled her and when he rang back he said it was probably thrush in the gullet.

Next day Benjamin left for Wellington to attend a course. He went to say goodbye to Rebecca. Her face fell. 'I wish he didn't have to leave,' she said.

While Chris took them to the airport, Prue, one of the district nurses, stayed with Rebecca and me. She wanted me to sleep, but I couldn't sit still, so I cleaned the house and did the washing. Finally I sat beside Prue at Rebecca's bedside, watching her breathing alternate between shallow little gasps, then deep rhythmic inhalations. I took Prue into my study and showed her a photo of Rebecca with Fabiano and Bruno, taken four years before. She admired her long, tanned legs. 'We don't often get to see them when they're like that,' she said.

Them?

I wished she hadn't said that.

I wished the ambulance officer hadn't said sympathetically on our return journey to Greendale one day, 'Poor thing. How long has she got?'

I'd put my finger to my lips to warn her into silence. She glanced at Rebecca lying with her eyes closed and bit her lip. 'Oh, I'm sorry,' she said. 'I didn't think.'

No.

I wished the doctor in ED hadn't told her when she'd had yet another bowel obstruction. 'It may clear itself. It may not. If it doesn't, that's it.'

Did these people grow an extra layer of skin to help them live with death? Was there something missing in their training? Or were they just naturally stupid?

Chris arrived back with a new, blue nightie for Rebecca. We put it on her. Her eyes were bright and she could speak clearly. To my delight she asked for some yoghurt and was able to swallow a little. Prue helped us get her back into the chair in the living room and then left.

At 7pm she fainted again when she tried to stand up to get back from the commode to the chair. This time black blood gushed out of her nose and mouth. 'Can't breathe,' she gasped, her eyes wide. We gave her some oxygen and she calmed down. I called John and Sue to come over and John called the nurses back. By the time they arrived her colour was better. She pushed everyone away and said she didn't want to feel anyone near her.

After a few minutes she smiled and reached out to touch each person, naming each one. She touched my cheek and said she couldn't see us very clearly, so needed to check who was in the room. When she'd identified everyone she asked who else had come through the door. I said it was probably one of the nurses. She shook her head. No, someone else had come in, but she couldn't see who it was. I said there was no one else there, just the seven of us. She looked puzzled and I asked if her vision was blurred. She said it was. She asked us to help her sit upright in the chair and began to talk animatedly to everyone. She was very interested in the conversation, and discussed a racehorse with John and told him she'd like to train a white horse when she got better.

Suddenly she turned to Mary and asked, 'What sound does a bear make when it's stung by a bee?'

We thought it was a riddle, but she said she didn't know the answer either. I asked her why she'd thought of it and she laughed and said she had no idea. She began to move her legs around restlessly and asked several times to be helped to sit upright. Then she began having pain in her abdomen and over about an hour the nurses gave her more morphine. The pain began to subside. John asked her if the experience she'd had earlier in the evening, of not being able to breathe, was scary and she said it was and asked him if he'd had personal experience of that. With the emphysema he'd been suffering from for the last five years he certainly had, and he described to her how he'd felt. I touched Rebecca's feet. They were very cold, so I began to massage them and asked if she'd like a head massage. She said she was okay and that she didn't feel at all cold.

The nurses decided to leave as she seemed much better. As they got ready to go I said to Rebecca, 'You gave me such a fright. I think I might have to spoil you a bit now.'

She grinned. 'I'm used to that.'

At 9.45 I said goodbye to them on the porch and they told me they couldn't believe how she kept rallying.

'She has a very strong will to live,' said Mary.

'It won't be much longer,' said Prue, trying to comfort me. 'Her skin has that dusky colour. That's a sign.'

This, of course, offered no comfort at all. 'There are always miracles,' I said.

They both agreed that indeed there were. I dried my tears and tried to compose myself before going back in the house, wondering how long Rebecca could keep on inhabiting her poor, devastated body. I knew she might not make it through the night. In spite of all her determination, courage and strength, as I walked back through the door I finally knew there would be no miracle.

# THIRTEEN

# Visit of the fantail

Rebecca's eyes were closed. Her face was snuggled into the soft leather of the chair. Sue said she'd just told Rebecca that she and John were staying with her for a few hours so we could get some sleep, and if she wanted anything to let them know. She'd smiled and thanked Sue then closed her eyes. As I sat down I saw Rebecca's chest was still. Chris came back into the living room with a cup of tea. He stared at Rebecca and looked at me. We moved close to her mouth and nose and felt the tiniest breath of air. Chris found a pulse in her neck beating very faintly. John and Sue said they'd wait outside on the verandah. Chris and I knelt by her chair.

We held her hands and told her how much we loved her and that she was now free to go and ride her white horse.

At 10.10 her pulse was gone.

Very calmly, I went out to the verandah to tell John and Sue and they said they knew because the wind had been blowing strongly and in the last two minutes there'd been complete stillness. I listened. Even the earth was holding its breath.

John phoned the nurses. They came back and with Chris, lifted Rebecca into the wheelchair and took her into her bedroom.

'Don't drop her,' I said.

Sue helped them wash her. There was no trace of the strong muscles, the golden skin radiating health, though one of the nurses told me her skin was in good condition, much better than she usually saw in cancer patients. I fretted that I hadn't cleaned her teeth that morning. The nurses assured me they'd done it now. I saw they'd taken the Fentanyl patch off her arm, and detached the morphine pump. That's right, I thought, she doesn't need them any more. They took off the ileostomy bag and put a plaster across the wound. At last it was off. Rebecca would be pleased. Mary asked if I wanted to comb her hair. It had grown back thick and soft and curly, though darker than it had been. I combed it with the pink brush Rebecca had used since she was six. We tucked her into her bed. Sing jumped on the bed, settled down and started purring.

I stroked Rebecca's still warm face.

All the treatment.

All the prayers.

All leading to this.

She left when we weren't looking.

She slipped out of the world as easily as she'd slipped into it.

No drama.

No fuss.

She was born.

She lived.

She died.

Rebecca has died.

Rebecca is dead.

Our child.

Dead.

Lying in her bed.

Dead in her bed.

Dead.

I walked into my study, stepped out of my skin, and watched myself looking at the photos on the wall. Rebecca. Playing ice hockey. Holding the goat. Arms around Fabiano and Bruno. A school photo.

Alive.

Then she was alive.

Golden.

Whole.

Her whole life in front of her.

Now she is dead.

But I was observing it all from a very great distance.

From this new detached perspective I watched myself pick up the phone and call Susannah and Benjamin.

Susannah said, 'But it *can't* be! Not *yet*! I was coming over tomorrow.'

I heard myself telling her to find Mark and drive on over. Mark was out at a movie so Susannah went to look for him. Later she told me that the doorman at the cinema wouldn't let her in. She explained her sister had just died and she needed to find her husband. He still wouldn't let her pass so she pushed him aside and ran into the cinema, calling for Mark. When they emerged, the place was swarming with security guards. She ignored them. 'They didn't try to stop me, Mum. I think they knew that if they tried I'd have to kill them.'

While we waited for Susannah and Mark, I cleared out all the boxes of morphine from the cupboards, all the needles and syringes, all the pills. Mary and Prue took them away. A few months later when I pulled out the oven to clean behind it I found a needle on the floor. The sight made me feel sick.

Susannah walked into Rebecca's room and burst into tears. She'd intended coming to visit the following day, she cried, so how could this have happened *now*?

Benjamin and Dee said they'd fly back with Elliot the next day. Dee told me that after Benjamin had put the phone down he'd gone into Elliot's bedroom and brought him into bed with them and wept.

I slept fitfully that night. I dreamt I saw Rebecca looking through a window at me, her face covered in tears. Chris said he'd heard her voice calling, 'Dad!' and felt a weight on the bed by his feet.

In the morning, in the fraction of a second before consciousness, I knew that there was something I needed to remember. Then, in full awareness, I ran into her room. I'd find that she'd simply been sleeping deeply and we'd mistakenly thought she'd died, just like that dream I had last year.

No.

She was lying in the same position in which we'd left her. I touched her cheek. Soft. Cool. But not cold. She had a little smile on her lips. Rebecca's cats came in. Sing jumped on the bed, stopped, stared, and tried to get into bed with her. Song stayed at the bottom of the bed. They looked at me. But I was already drifting out of my skin again.

A locum GP from Darfield arrived to certify Rebecca's death. I took him to her room and left him there. When he came out he mentioned to Chris that his sister was doing an engineering course at Canterbury University and started chatting cheerily about the university. I stared at him in disbelief, but yet again, I stayed silent.

As I look back on this and similar situations during Rebecca's illness and after her death, I wonder why I didn't speak my mind. I believe it was because the territory was so foreign that I had no language with which to negotiate it. Although I was certainly aware of my feelings of outrage that thoughtless words and behaviour gave rise to, I simply had no words to express these feelings. Instead I questioned whether I'd heard correctly. I told myself I must have misunderstood, that nobody could be so stupid, that I should not make a scene in case I'd got it all wrong and ended up embarrassing the undoubtedly well-meaning, but misguided, person who'd upset me.

Two weeks later when Chris fell off Jade and the ambulance stopped at the Darfield surgery for the paperwork before taking him to hospital, that same locum was there and wanted me to go into the surgery to sign forms. My grey face? My tears? The semi-conscious man on the stretcher? FORMS? I told him the forms could wait. We. Needed. To. Get. Chris. To. Hospital. NOW.

In the following years my tolerance of such crassness shrank to zero.


The morning after Rebecca died, whatever energy had been holding me up and directing my steps suddenly drained away. In the middle of a sentence I was left directionless, wordless, skinless, stripped back to the bone. I screamed. And screamed and screamed and screamed and screamed and screamed. The screaming turned into wailing and the wailing turned into a sound I'd never heard before. I found out later the word for it was keening. The keening went on and on and on until there was no more breath. Chris and Susannah held me and wept.

I extracted myself from their arms and walked to the window overlooking the rose garden where, just 18 months ago, we'd buried Momma's ashes. I remembered the little fantail that Susannah and Rebecca had seen flitting from branch to branch, watching us. Piwakawaka. The messenger. I drifted into my study and stood wondering what I'd gone in there for. A fantail came right up to the window, tapped on it and looked at me. I called Chris. It flew away. When he stood beside me it returned to look at him.

The undertakers, both women, arrived and wheeled a coffin in the front door. I took one look at it and started walking in circles around the room. 'No no no no no no no no no no no no no no …'

From somewhere far away I heard one of them say to Chris, 'It's all right. Just let her pace like that. Don't try and stop her.'

They took the coffin into Rebecca's room. Mark helped them lift Rebecca into it. We went to look at her lying in the coffin, her hands folded together. Her beautiful long artist's fingers. Kevin's voice, two years ago, telling me about his son's motorbike accident. *'When yer see yer own son lyin' in his coffin it rips yer heart out.'* Rebecca, nodding her head. *'Yeah. I can imagine.'*

But back then we couldn't.

Susannah fretted that she didn't look comfortable. We should wrap her up in a warm blanket.

'It's all right. She's not there any more,' I said.

We placed photographs of family and friends, soft toys that people had brought her while she was ill, and some horse ornaments she'd loved around her chest. I put a little white silk horse in her hands. It was one of a set of six we'd used as Christmas tree ornaments for many years and the previous Christmas Rebecca had asked if she could keep them in her room. She'd given a red one to Fabiano as a gift before he left last week.

Bart arrived later in the morning. As he came through the front door he said, 'Hey, the weirdest thing. As I got out of the car a fantail circled round me all the way up to the door.'

Then Natasha arrived. I took Bart and her into Rebecca's room. They stood in silence, tears running down their faces, touching Rebecca's hands. Bart told the story of the fantail to Natasha and at the same moment a fantail tapped at the window, looking at Natasha. When John and Sue arrived they said a fantail had come to their window that morning.

Susannah said, 'Mum, Rebecca's telling us she's free.'

Benjamin and Dee and Elliot arrived. Benjamin told me he didn't want to see Rebecca dead. I knew he was thinking of the awful picture Momma had presented in death. Rebecca didn't look like that, I assured him. But he was adamant.

On Monday morning Fabiano rang from Brazil. He'd been driving back home when his mother had phoned to tell him Rebecca had died. He'd driven all the way back to Belo Horizonte where his mother and sister waited up for him till he arrived. I told him about the fantail. At that moment a fantail tapped at my bedroom window. We were both in tears as I related this. I asked him what he'd like me to say on his behalf at Rebecca's funeral that afternoon.

'Say that she made me feel very alive every time I was with her,' he said.

We couldn't face a large, formal funeral. All of Rebecca's friends from Art School were away on end of term holidays and I had no energy to try and contact them. Nor did we want to have her body embalmed, which a delayed funeral would have made necessary. After all the poking and prodding she'd endured in the last year I wanted no stranger's hand touching her in death. We invited only her closest friends to gather in our garden at 1pm that afternoon.

Chris, Benjamin and Mark swept away the autumn leaves on the lawn in front of Rebecca's room and set out chairs. They brought the coffin out onto the verandah in front of her bedroom and covered it with a horse blanket, saddle, her riding hat and boots. We put hay bales in front of it and arranged her ice hockey boots, her paint palettes and brushes and flowers on them. Benjamin took charge of the music. He played Rebecca's favourite, from *Braveheart*, as everyone arrived.

Chris welcomed everyone and slowly and steadily talked about Rebecca's growing up years. Benjamin spoke about their childhood and how much she'd meant to him as a playmate and a friend. I was so proud of how he spoke and what he said. Then I told everyone what Fabiano had asked me to say that morning when he'd phoned. Benjamin played the track from a U2 CD, *Who's Gonna Ride your Wild Horses?* that Fabiano had said, four years ago, expressed his feelings about Rebecca when he was so in love with her and she didn't want him. Bart and Grant spoke about their exploits at school and the time they'd brought their old car to our garden and spray painted it, and the fun they'd all had every weekend that the car was here.

Finally we played 'Time to Say Goodbye' by Andrea Bocelli, from the Romanza CD, which was also one of Rebecca's favourites. John brought over a tiny rowan sapling from his garden. We planted it near Fabiano's Tree where it would grow to overlook the paddocks and mountains. On Rebecca's 24th birthday, the following month, we would bury her ashes there.

We all went indoors and ate food prepared by our neighbours and friends and they looked at Rebecca's artwork and photographs, which we'd arranged on the table. Several people said they'd seen a fantail sitting on a branch, watching the whole proceedings.

Kevin started telling me about the time Rebecca had worked on his farm and her daring in the way she trained horses. She refused to give up, he said, no matter how many times they bucked her off, until she had them eating out of her hand. As I was listening to this story the undertakers arrived.

Benjamin, Bart, Grant and Mark carried the coffin into the hearse. Chris and I walked behind. When it was in the hearse I leaned over the coffin until Chris led me away, supporting me in his arms as the hearse slowly drove from our home to begin its journey to the crematorium. Six years later Kevin told me that in all his 77 years, this was the saddest sight he'd ever seen.

By evening everyone had gone, except Susannah and Mark, Benjamin, Dee and Elliot. Benjamin talked about the fantail Dee had seen in Rebecca's room a year ago. The tohu. Impending death. Chris said he didn't believe in that. Fantails came in and out of the house on a fairly regular basis. 'And the rest of us are still here, aren't we?'

But still.

We talked about the things people had said and how deeply moved we'd been to realise the ways in which Rebecca had touched their lives. I hadn't been able to imagine how we'd face what we'd faced in the last few days, but we had. And I was glad she'd slipped away quietly and peacefully, without any fear, surrounded by her family, in her own home, and that her appalling suffering was finally at an end. Nonetheless, how we would be able to live in a world without Rebecca was not at all clear.

# FOURTEEN

# Ashes

A fantail sat in the ivy on the barn and watched as we packed the wheelchair and commode into the car. Chris drove into town to return them to the hospital. He came home with Rebecca's ashes. Before he had time to move them to his study I walked into the laundry and saw a small, green cardboard box on the washing machine. On the side it read *Cremains of Rebecca Elizabeth Arnold*. I looked from the box to the sink where, only two years ago, she'd stood washing her pet ferret, Stinky. Bare-footed, in shorts and crop top, eyes sparkling, grinning at the camera, with the soapy ferret draped over her hands like a piece of stretchy rubber. Now she no longer had a body. Her beautiful smile, her talents, her hopes and dreams all fitted into this small green box. This was beyond tears. This was beyond my ability to stay in my skin.

Over the following week I launched into a maniacal cleaning frenzy. The house shone, inside and out. Next we started on the garden, pruning trees, letting the light in. We worked in the paddocks in the rain from morning till night, clearing the trimmings from the gorse hedge that had just been cut and loading them onto the bonfire and burning them along with all the other garden rubbish. A contractor came to cut back the two huge macrocarpa trees in the paddock, Chris sawed up the logs into firewood for the winter and I heaved them into the wheelbarrow and trundled them to the woodshed. It was hard physical work, but we needed to have a reason to stay out of the house all day so we could be exhausted enough to fall asleep at night. Even so, sleep was fitful and racked with terrifying dreams. Waking in the morning was worse. Always the split second of forgetfulness followed by an awareness of something that needed to be remembered. Then full consciousness that left me breathless, hollowed out, scraped raw.

Friends visited with flowers and food and company. They invited us out, but we couldn't face rejoining the world. We talked about selling the house and leaving the area, but had no energy to begin such a process. People phoned and asked how we were, but I had no words to express how we were. We avoided sitting at the table to eat because the empty place was more intensely redolent of Rebecca than ever her physical presence had been, though she'd rarely sat at the table with us in those last few weeks. When the food ran out I started to cook again and decided to set the table. Only when we sat down did I realise I'd set it for three.

It exhausted me to answer the phone or receive visitors. However, I recognised that other people loved Rebecca and had a need to come to our home and grieve too. Sometimes I was surprised by the intensity of their grief. Sometimes I had to be the one who gave comfort.

A week after Rebecca died we left the house to go to Mark's graduation ceremony at the Christchurch Town Hall. He asked Chris to go on stage with the other academics. Chris felt he couldn't face that, but he compromised by bringing his gown to the graduation so he and Mark could have photographs taken together. However, as we took our seats in the auditorium Chris said he regretted his decision not to go on stage. He looked for the organiser and asked for an extra chair to be put there so he could take part. Afterwards we went with Susannah, Mark, Melanie, his parents and aunt to the Curator's House in the Botanic Gardens for lunch. It was a day of celebration. But it didn't feel real.

Two weeks after Rebecca died I saw in the TV guide that *Xena: Warrior Princess* was on that evening. Rebecca had loved the series and said Xena was her role model. Though I normally didn't watch it, I felt the need to watch this one. The episode concluded with Xena's death and her reappearance to her friend, Gabrielle. She assured Gabrielle that she would always be there for her in spirit. I wept and said to Chris, 'I didn't know it was the final. I thought Xena was indestructible.'

Our GP, Peter Law, came to see us the day he got back from Europe. He was of the generation of doctors who considered home visits normal. When my children were growing up he told me to call him any time of day or night that I was concerned about them. Coming from England where doctors barely bothered to raise their heads from their prescription pads during a consultation, I found his manner warm, engaging, and infinitely reassuring as I brought up my children in a country far from home and family.

He was in tears as I described Rebecca's last days and the funeral ceremony and the fantail. After listening to this he said he was glad he'd made the trip to see us. For years after Rebecca's birth, whenever I'd taken her to see him, he'd laughingly ascribed her childhood ailments to the fact she'd 'been born in a cave', referring to the Leboyer birthing method of having the lights dimmed. Just before she died he told Chris he wanted to be the one who certified her death. But just as he'd missed her entrance into the world so too had he missed her exit.

The district nurses, Mary and Prue, called in to see me. At the same time Kate, the palliative care doctor, rang up. When I told them about the fantail they all said that they believed Rebecca's spirit was so strong she'd have found a way to send us some comfort after her death and that because of her affinity with nature, sending the fantail was the way she'd do it. They also said she was able to die in the way she had, without fear or pain, because of all the love around her. A few days later, the stoma care nurse, who'd been so abrupt about Rebecca's minding the ileostomy bag, rang and said the same thing. She sounded kind. I wished she'd been kinder to Rebecca.

Some friends brought over nine white rose bushes – one from each of them. We planted them in the rose garden. Another friend brought a white camellia which we planted near the rowan tree, opposite Rebecca's bedroom window.

Natasha and Bart came out and spent the whole day with us. They wanted to talk and talk about Rebecca. Bart was in tears. He said he couldn't believe she was gone and still couldn't accept it, 'Even when I saw Becks in that coffin.' Someone he knew had attempted suicide. This made him angry because Rebecca wanted so much to live. Natasha regretted the two years she'd spent in Australia when she could have been with Rebecca. They spoke about the things they'd done with Rebecca at high school and the parties they'd gone to. Most of the tales I hadn't heard before and I enjoyed hearing about the crazy things they'd done and the fun they'd all had. They went through the photograph albums and selected some photographs of them all together. We promised to get copies made.

Fabiano wrote about his distress that he wasn't there when Rebecca died. I told him that Chris had said Rebecca couldn't leave while he and all her friends and her brother and sister were there. That they all needed to leave before she could.

Sue said she was overcome by grief one day and couldn't stop crying. That night when she went to bed she dreamt that Rebecca was standing at the foot of the bed in her riding clothes, smiling and happy. The next day Sue went for a ride on Red and decided to take him for a ride every day.

I went out into the paddock to groom the horses and set out jumping poles. I sat on the barrels Rebecca had placed under a couple of trees. With my eyes closed I tried to hear the sounds of cantering hooves and pictured Rebecca, long, blonde hair flying out behind her as she took the horse towards the jump. 'Did ya see that, Mum?' But I opened my eyes to empty spaces and silence.

Chris wandered out to find me and I asked him whether he thought it was best to die quickly in an accident, with no time to say goodbye, or die by inches, as Rebecca had, even though we did have time to say all the things we wanted to. He didn't know. Then John and Sue came over and Chris brought cups of tea into the paddock. As we stood talking, Chris jumped onto Jade's back. It was something Rebecca had done many times. However, it was a terrible error of judgement on Chris's part because Jade hadn't been ridden bareback for months. Not only that, Chris had never learned to ride. I was about to tell him to get off and Sue was about to go for a bridle, when Jade trotted off, gathering speed. Chris tried to jump off, but fell to the ground, landing on his head.

We ran over to him. He was white, his pupils had dilated and his pulse was weak. He didn't know where he was or what had happened. John called the ambulance while I sat by Chris, wailing. Just before Chris was lifted into the ambulance his memory returned briefly and with it, the memory of Rebecca's death, as if he'd heard it for the first time. In the ambulance he drifted off, woke up to ask what had happened and again and again cried, 'She's dead, isn't she?'

Sue came with me to the hospital, her calm, reassuring presence preventing me from lapsing into hysteria. The trip to hospital, the ED, the same doctors and nurses, were all a nightmarish replay of recent months. Fortunately, it turned out Chris wasn't seriously injured and after four hours he was discharged. When we arrived home the fire was on and a meal was in the oven, prepared by John.

The incident was yet another reminder of the precarious hold we had on life. The world no longer felt safe or predictable. Susannah was devastated by Rebecca's death and had started thinking of having a baby to ensure life's continuity. Benjamin left the Church. He said he no longer wanted to sing about the grace of God when there was no grace to be found in his sister dying at the age of 23.

I knew that when Rebecca graduated she'd leave home to go travelling or flatting and I wanted to savour her company as long as we had her with us. She'd told me many months before she was diagnosed with cancer that she longed to travel, but that ultimately she would want to buy land near us. 'I just can't imagine myself living far away from you and Dad,' she said, and I'd laughed, thinking of the teacher having to prise her little, white-knuckled fingers off my hand the day she started school. Little limpet was our nickname for her. But this was no normal nest-emptying.

There were Rebecca-shaped spaces everywhere we looked. Her paintings hung on the walls and filled her room. Her clothes hung in her cupboard. Her dog and cats and horses and goat still needed to be taken care of and fed. We heard the same sounds she'd loved, the stags roaring at night, the wind in the trees, the horses whinnying in the paddocks. But within these objects and animals and within these sounds there were no gales of laughter. No wood cuttings littered the floor, no paint-stained cloths on the table, no half-eaten sandwiches on the bench. I could smell her scent on her hairbrush and her clothes – summer grass, saturated with sun. I could hear her voice in my head. But oh, the silence. Oh, the stillness.

We sat down to have dinner, but I couldn't stop crying. I didn't know where to go or what to do. Then suddenly the thought came to me to go and groom the horses.

'What … *now?*' said Chris.

'Yes, now.' I said.

Their smell. Their warm breath on my head as I picked out their hooves and brushed their manes. This was exactly what Rebecca had done when she was sad. It was the best form of therapy that existed, in her opinion. And she was right. I stopped crying and hugged the horses. And thought of her jumping over the gate at the end of a ride, washing their tack, brushing them, putting their rugs on as I called, 'I'll run you a bath and start dinner.'

Another day when I was working in the paddocks, I thought of stories people had told me of sensing their dead relatives near them: an unexpected whiff of perfume, the radio unaccountably turning on, a light touch on the side of the head. My father had told me that when he was dozing in a chair a few days after my mother died, he felt a soft pressure on his foot and woke to see her sitting opposite him smiling. 'It only lasted a few seconds,' he said, 'and then she was gone. But I know she was there. I wasn't dreaming.' Well, if it gives him comfort to think that, we'd said. I remembered that he'd been extremely scathing of my aunt's involvement in spiritualism. The dead do not return, he insisted. Only in dreams. His own beloved sister had returned to him many times in dreams after she'd died of peritonitis in her late twenties.

My brother told me our mother's favourite flower had bloomed at her front door.

'Coincidence,' we said.

'Probably,' he agreed. 'But in winter?'

My longing to have Rebecca with me again, to see her and touch her, filled me with despair far beyond tears. Beyond my ability to express in any way whatsoever. My grief was physical and my whole body ached as I walked over to the trench she had dug in one of the paddocks so she could train Jade to get over his fear of jumping ditches. I called her name. Let the wind carry her name. A sheep from the neighbouring paddock bleated loudly in response. It sounded distressed and I saw it was trapped with its head stuck in the fence. I pulled at the fence, but I couldn't free it.

Oh, stupid sheep.

Wire-cutters! Go *on*!

Where?

In the *shed*!

What do wire-cutters look like?

*These* ones *here*! In the *toolbox*!

I cut the wire and the sheep pulled its head free. It stopped and looked at me and gave a grunt before running off.

'You're welcome,' I called after it. What had I expected? That Rebecca would waft by me playing a harp?

Get *real*, Mum!

An email arrived from my friend John in Australia:

> *The way you have written about Rebecca's death is a gift. For me, for I feel you*
> *have included me in your family's experience. For anyone else with whom you*
> *share this treasure. For yourself, because language as an exploration and assertion*
> *of consciousness is a shining thread through the darkness. Perhaps also for Rebecca*
> *whose being and consciousness undoubtedly will have participated in the act of*
> *writing. Somehow, the challenge now to live in the enormity of everyday grief and*
> *to simultaneously imagine that other perspective, in which all meanings cohere, is*
> *to be met, and I know you have the strength to accomplish this.*

Six years from then he would experience the pain of watching his second wife battle with cancer at the same time as his first wife, the mother of his children, died from it.

The first time I went to the supermarket I automatically picked up the food Rebecca liked. That reminded me she would never eat again and I almost fled. The first trip to the mall horrified me. The glare. The noise. The packs of people. I could hardly breathe and left as soon as I could. After a month, Chris went back to work. He rang me to say he was driving home with the radio on and started singing, then with the realisation that he was singing, a wave of sorrow hit him so hard he had to pull over to the side of the road.

A week before Rebecca's birthday on 9 May, we began sorting through her artwork. Some of it we put aside to frame. Others, a few heads of female warriors, we selected to give to Sari, Susannah's friend, who wanted to make cards with them. Looking at all Rebecca's drawings again reminded us how talented she was and how much she was able to cram into her short life.

My days were spent taking care of the horses. They were in John's paddock and I went over there every day to feed them. Each time I did this I was in tears. 'Think of the good times,' people advised. But I couldn't bear to think of the times we'd ridden together and the times I'd watched Rebecca's rapport with these beautiful animals that she'd walked among, bare-footed. Sometimes John and Sue were in the paddock and saw my tears. They didn't try to tell me everything would be okay, that it was God's will, that time heals, that God needed her more than I did, that I was lucky I had two other children, or any of the other well-meaning but idiotic clichés we'd heard over recent weeks. They simply let me cry and speak her name.

I couldn't keep four horses, so I contacted Darryn and asked him to sell Bug and Kit for me. I thought it would break my heart to see Bug and Kit go, but I reminded myself that Rebecca would trust Darryn to find them a good home. I would keep Red because he was old and Rebecca had promised him he'd stay with us all his life and I'd keep Jade and ride him. I oiled all the bridles and washed the saddle blankets and started working with Jade. I had both horses wormed and shod and their teeth filed, and rang the physiotherapist to come and check their backs and legs. The saddles were due for their annual check. When the saddler came out he said the horses were looking great and where was Rebecca?

'She died.'

'You're kidding!'

I shook my head.

His face fell. 'But … she was a *gorgeous* girl!'

'Yes. She was.'

9 May, Rebecca's 24th birthday.

We invited Natasha, Grant, Bart, John and Sue to join our family. Benjamin gave them a booklet he'd designed on the computer, with two pictures of Rebecca. One showed her riding Red; the other was cut from a photo of Benjamin and Susannah standing next to Rebecca on her 23rd birthday. She was wearing the oilskin riding coat I'd given her that day. At 4pm we all went out into the garden.

*Chris puts the green box on the earth next to the rowan tree. 'Rowan, protector of young women,' Rebecca had said, filing sketches for her Celtic Goddess project. We reach into the box and take a handful of ashes. A truck hurtles down the gravel road, shattering the stillness, sending up clouds of dust. There's no wind yet, but later there'll be gusts, scattering red and gold leaves around the garden. We need to say her name, but we have no breath. I form its shape in silence. Let her name float on the wind. Let it drift like mist around the verandah posts, under the eaves of the house, in and out of the trees and bushes, over the paddocks where the sheep graze, down the road to the river, where the Alps shine against a brilliant blue, where the tracks are covered in orange poppies and wild purple lupins, where the air is filled with the humming of bees and the songs of larks, and the striking of hooves on stone. And the girl on the horse turns. She flicks back her long blonde hair. And looks at you with eyes as blue as the sky.*

*The ashes slip through our fingers to the roots of the rowan. I wonder why they're called ashes. They're not. They're grit. Pure grit.*

I didn't know how I was going to face seeing our beautiful daughter reduced to ashes. But I needed to feel them in my hand because that was the last time I could touch part of her. One by one the others came up and did the same, including Elliot, now aged 20 months. Benjamin was the only one who used the trowel. He couldn't bear to touch his sister's ashes. When we'd finished we all put sprigs of rosemary on top of the ashes. Chris sprinkled in some horse poo. A strange symbol, but it felt right. We filled in the hole with soil then stood up and looked around. To my astonishment the world hadn't stopped spinning.

We went back into the house and had dinner together. In the centre of the table I had placed a structure that Rebecca had made the previous year as an art project to represent her past and present life. It was a small wooden staircase, on one side of which she'd stuck a collage of black and white photographs of her childhood, and on the other, coloured photographs representing her present life, all including horses. On each step of the stair I placed objects that were special to her. On the top step I laid a yellow rose from the bush that bloomed over Momma's ashes.

I described this day to a friend who'd lost his baby daughter many years before. Jim replied:

> *Two things struck me. One was the tremendous importance of ceremony and our human need to give significance to the moment by special words, special actions, special music and the gathering together of items with symbolic importance. I feel we live in an age that often turns its back on ceremony and we are often left inadequate when the need for it is there. Of course, ceremony can become frozen and stultified and lose its charge, ritualistically gone through when there is no real cause for it. But it seems you were able to reinvest the moment with simple forms and tremendous meaning. Of course, it would have been exhausting, but necessary, and terribly sad, and beautiful. The other thing you mentioned was the astonishment that the ordinary world seems to go on, that the sky did not turn green, that some people and creatures were sublimely unaware that something monumental had taken place and was taking place. That for you, and for Rebecca, the world had changed forever. I remember when Zoe died finding it hard to accept that the man riding his bike along the street could do so at all, could pedal past our gate in a state of not-knowing.*

Not knowing could be forgiven, I thought. But by now I'd begun to wonder about those who did know and yet continued on their way past the gate, either literally or metaphorically.

# FIFTEEN

# Empty spaces

In June I was ready to return to work. Before Chris dropped me off I began to weep and said I couldn't face going in. He drove around the block a few times until I felt able to walk through the door. As I walked into the building one of my colleagues saw me. She came over and held me for a moment before leading me to my new office. She explained that they thought I'd feel better in a smaller office with three other people, rather than being in the large teachers' room. I went into the teachers' room to find my files and suddenly there were hands all around me, picking up my files, carrying them to my office, touching my arm. The Head of School came in and welcomed me back. Beginning again was easier than I'd thought.

Though I was dreading facing a class, I found it was possible to keep my mind focused on teaching my students and in so doing, my grief could move to one side for a while. However, as soon as I got in the car to drive home the lump in my chest began to swell until my tears fell in torrents.

I avoided driving by the shop where Rebecca bought her art supplies, or crossing the road where she and I used to cross together before she turned into the Art and Design School and I turned into my own building, waving and calling, 'Have a good day. See you later.' One afternoon, however, I felt a strong urge to drive by the art supplies shop. I pulled in to the side of the road where I used to wait for Rebecca until she came out laden with coloured card, more brushes, a new craft knife. I thought of her passion for ice hockey and the poster she'd made advertising women's ice hockey: ***Break some ice. Chill out. Be cool.***

Floods of tears.

A bus passed.

On the back was a poster advertising Alpine Ice Rink.

**CHILL OUT. BE COOL. SKATE AT ALPINE.**

I stared.

A car overtook the bus.

On the number plate, **BECKS.**

I walked over to the Art and Design School to collect a model stable Rebecca had made as an advertising project for perfume. The Head of Department told me how shocked he and the staff still felt. 'I expected a knock at my door and Rebecca standing there saying she was ready to start again,' he said, tears in his eyes as he handed over the model.

Back at my desk I opened the roof of the stable and took out three little perfume bottles nestled in hay. Rebecca had called the perfume *Equidae* and each bottle had a label affixed: *Feel. Timing. Balance.* These were the principles of horse riding that Darryn had taught her. I would write to him and let him know, I thought, unscrewing the cap of *Feel*. As the familiar scent was released, my throat ached. A couple of colleagues walked down the passage outside my office, talking animatedly and laughing. The photocopier groaned. A cup rattled in a saucer. Someone sighed over a pile of essays. I wanted to be somewhere else, but I didn't know where. Yes, I did. Burje.

Burje had propped Rebecca's painting against the wall of his living room. I looked at the vibrant colours and the pale face in profile and told him I'd interpreted the vortex as Rebecca's reaction to the appalling situation she was caught up in. He replied that he and Bronwyn had interpreted it as a tunnel of light and the fact that the face was in profile and poised at the edge of the tunnel showed that Rebecca was poised between life and death at the time of painting it. Since then I've seen several paintings by Maori of the same spiral pattern representing birth, life, death and rebirth.

Susannah rang me to say she'd been lying in bed that morning thinking about Rebecca and wondering how she felt as she died. The next moment she appeared to be looking down on our house in Greendale and saw Rebecca lying in bed. As she drew closer she dreaded seeing Rebecca's dead body. Suddenly she realised she was looking down on herself, asleep in her own bed. With that realisation she awoke in her body.

'I think Rebecca was showing me what it was like for her,' she said.

During a medical check-up I burst into tears. My 10-minute consultation turned into 40 minutes as Joy, my gynecologist, listened to me. She told me how she'd felt when her father died when she was young and she drew a circle on a piece of paper.

'This is your life. And this,' drawing another circle that enclosed the first, 'is your grief. It completely fills your life now. As you start adding other layers to your life this is what happens.' She drew bigger circles around the original one. 'You see what happens? Your grief stays the same. It doesn't decrease in size. But your life will grow around it.'

This made the most sense that I'd ever heard and I thanked her while apologising for taking so much of her time.

'I take the time it takes,' she said.

At the end of June we travelled to Wellington to stay with Benjamin, Dee and Elliot for a few days. This was the first time we'd been away from home since we'd taken Rebecca to Auckland. It was unsettling being in a landscape that didn't even hold the empty spaces that the Canterbury one now did.

While we were in the North Island, the South Island was gripped by arctic weather. Nine inches of snow fell in Greendale, which cut off the electricity for 24 hours and brought down trees. On our arrival home we went out to inspect the damage in our garden.

Shredded trees and flattened shrubs lay strewn around the sodden garden, but the worst damage was to the big old plum tree. Its spreading branches had provided a cool, shady umbrella in the hot Canterbury summers. It attracted blackbirds and thrushes and fantails and silver-eyes and goldfinches, and that part of the garden was always filled with their singing. On summer evenings I used to sling a hammock between this tree and a cherry tree and lie in it, reading the paper. Invariably Rebecca would find me there and hop in beside me, first grabbing a handful of juicy, purple plums we could munch on as we chatted about our day and made plans for the next horse trek. The snowstorm had torn off the branch the hammock had been tied to, leaving a great gaping hole in the trunk. The saturated tree was partially uprooted and leaned towards the earth. We stared at it in dismay.

'It won't survive,' Chris said.

Against all odds, it did.

Grant sent us an invitation to his engagement party at the end of June. We thanked him, but explained we weren't yet up to attending social gatherings. I told him that Rebecca had always said he and Kirsten made a great couple. Engagements. Weddings. Babies. All these would happen to her friends in the coming years and I was glad of it. But still.

Chris and I spent a weekend sorting through everything in Rebecca's cupboards and desk. Some things could go in the attic. Some could stay in her cupboard. We packed away her music. I couldn't bear to listen to it again. Interspersed between the pages of the diary I'd given her when we went to Brazil were cartoons she'd collected from newspapers and translated into English. On one page she'd drawn a map with a heart marking Christchurch and the words: *Here lies my home. Always and forever.* I read the notes in her art books and laughed at the way she described her likes and dislikes. I enjoyed seeing the growing awareness and artistic development evident in these notes. Chris couldn't bear to read them.

I found some ultrasound film from November 1998 which was taken after Rebecca had consulted a doctor in Darfield because of pain in her abdomen. The ultrasound report stated there was nothing abnormal to be seen and no cause for the pain was found. I wondered now if the pain was caused by the tumour in her appendix. If her appendix had been examined then would she still be alive? If her appendix had been taken out when her ovary was removed, she wouldn't have suffered peritonitis and the hated ileostomy.

If only. If only. If only.

'I said it was her appendix,' fumed Burje. 'Why didn't they listen?'

Chris's sabbatical leave was due the following year. We'd planned on going to Brazil again when Rebecca graduated and she was planning to travel there herself. She wanted to spend some time on David's farm and was keen to see the progress of his riding school. She also planned on travelling to England to see her uncle, aunt and cousins and then travel through Ireland to explore the Celtic history she so loved. I dreaded the thought of the shadows we'd find in Brazil.

In July I started teaching my new course. Teaching forced a structure back into my daily routine that resembled normality. However, as I walked about the campus I half expected Rebecca to suddenly appear round a corner asking if I wanted to have lunch with her. But there'd be no more lunch time get-togethers. She wouldn't be coming home with me in the evenings.

The school counsellor popped her head around the door of my office and asked how things were going. I started to answer then lost my voice. I shook my head. She apologised and left. It took an hour to recover. Another day I went to the coffee room and overheard someone joking about how uplifting it was to attend a funeral. I knew my anger was irrational. I knew she wasn't aware I was standing behind her. I knew the best thing I could do was keep silent. But for a long time afterwards I couldn't bear the sight of this woman, or the sound of her braying laugh.

I had my two-yearly mammogram and had to be recalled for further assessment because of a shadow on the scan. I was shocked and Chris was beside himself with fear. Fortunately, further investigations revealed that there was nothing abnormal. Up until that scare I'd been thinking sometimes that life was too hard because I missed Rebecca so much it hurt to be alive. Then, when there was a possibility that my life might be shortened I realised I still wanted to be in the world. There were still things I needed to do. Not wanting to live without Rebecca was not the same as wanting to die. The false alarm, together with Chris's near fatal accident on the horse, was a turning point for both of us that forced us to appreciate the fact that we still had each other and two healthy children. We still had choices and still had our lives to live.

The Head of School announced she was resigning to go to Oman to establish a new English language school. She'd already been over to the Gulf and showed the staff some photos she'd taken. She asked us to let her know if anyone was interested in teaching there. I discussed with her the possibility of my teaching in Oman for a year and she was enthusiastic about the idea. Chris was less keen, but conceded that it might be better to go somewhere completely different rather than face the people and places in Brazil that had so enchanted us eight years ago.

One morning, driving to work, I was mulling over the pros and cons of going to Oman and fretting about leaving Susannah and Benjamin for an entire year when a bus pulled out in front of me. It had an advert for the Alpine Ice Rink on the back. On the bus advert there were three skaters: an ice hockey player, a speed skater and a figure skater. In large black letters the advert urged me to **Go hard! Go fast! Go figure! GO! GO! GO!**

Darina rang me to invite me to a seminar on death and dying. There would be a speaker, a doctor, who'd been trained by Elisabeth Kübler-Ross. The other speaker was a channel.

'A channel?'

'Just come and listen to him, Sandra. I know it's only been a month, but you might be ready.'

I thought of Deidre and Robert and all the others, the loopy-but-nice, the earnest-but-deluded, and the-ones-who-knew-they-were-charlatans that we'd wasted so much time and energy on over the past year and was about to say no. Instead, I said yes. That yes changed my life.

The death and dying seminar was held in Riccarton House, an old colonial home built by the Deans family 150 years ago. Many of the people attending were counsellors. Their chatter and laughter in the hall grated on me and I wandered away, pretending to examine the stuffed caribou heads mounted on the walls of the oak-panelled hall. These heads were the reason Rebecca objected so strenuously to us holding Susannah's wedding reception here six years before. No amount of persuasion that they were part of an earlier, less environmentally aware era could move her, so we'd chosen another venue.

I took my place with the other seminar participants in the old ballroom and the doctor, a gentle, elderly woman, spoke about the stages of grief. The second speaker was a man in his late thirties called Blair. He told us he channelled a being called Tabaash who'd lived 3000 years ago. We shouldn't be surprised, he said, to find that Tabaash had a sense of humour when he spoke to us about the stages of dying and the survival of the spirit. I stifled a sigh and wondered how quickly I could leave.

In the coffee break I went outside and sat by myself. Others approached me and told me of their losses. An adult son killed two years ago. A teenage son killed four years ago. A young daughter five years ago. They asked me why I was there. I told them. Only a month? Oh. It must have been very hard to leave the house and come here? Another woman sat beside me and introduced herself. She told me that her 19-year-old daughter had gone to England for her OE and had been diagnosed with cancer. She'd gone to England to bring her home. The pain was not well controlled and her daughter sank into a deep depression. One night she woke up and knew something felt wrong. She went to her daughter's room and found it empty. She went out into the garden and found her hanging from a tree.

'And you survived that?' I asked, in disbelief.

'It happened five years ago,' she said. 'I had to walk past that tree every day until it held no more horror for me.'

Blair was walking towards us, still channelling Tabaash. He came straight to me and said he had to give me a hug. I didn't want hugs from strangers, but as he approached I began to weep.

He said, 'She's with her soul group now. They're looking after her. She's still confused. Happy, but confused and trying to come to terms with what happened, because she had so many plans for the future and suddenly found the rug pulled out from under her.'

I listened and said nothing.

'She needs time to adjust to the new situation. She's around you a lot. You can talk to her. Play her music again. She had a lot of music. You didn't need to pack it away.'

When he left, the woman with me told me there was someone called Yasmeen, in Christchurch, doing the same sort of work. She worked with an entity called Raman. 'She gets very busy, however,' she warned, writing down the contact number. 'You might have to wait a few weeks.'

Next morning, as we were going into the seminar again, she came to apologise for telling me about her daughter. That must have made me feel even worse, she said, when my own grief was so new, so raw. I told her it didn't make me feel worse. It made me think that if she could survive seeing her daughter hanging from a tree, then I too might find a way to survive.

In the coffee break three elderly women arrived and peremptorily demanded to enter the house. Blair, still channelling Tabaash, said there was a seminar on death and dying going on, but they would be most welcome. They gasped and left hurriedly.

A young woman said, 'Imagine the look on their faces if you'd told them they were speaking to someone who was three thousand years old.'

Tabaash roared with laughter and I couldn't help laughing too.

Yasmeen's number lay on my desk for a week. I had no intention of ringing her. I'd met more than enough frauds during Rebecca's illness to last me a lifetime. Then one morning, on impulse, I rang the number. A pleasant female voice answered the phone and I asked if I could make an appointment. Yasmeen said she'd just that minute put the phone down on a cancellation for an appointment the next day. She could fit me in then if I liked.

Yasmeen walked into the waiting room. Early forties, tall with shiny auburn hair and bright blue, piercing eyes. Her skin was radiantly clear and her smile welcomed me warmly. She led me into her room, furnished with comfortable chairs and a low coffee table on which candles burned near a Buddha statuette. She indicated where I could sit and she sat opposite, explaining that she'd close her eyes and after a minute or so Raman would come through. I could ask him any questions I liked. Soon after she closed her eyes, her breathing deepened. She raised her head, still with closed eyes, and a male voice spoke.

The voice was that of a kindly old man.

'Salaam to you, my dearest heart. Welcome indeed. I am Raman and it is my pleasure to be here in support of your life, your journey, yourself ...'

To lose a child was a very hard thing for a mother to bear, he said. I hadn't given Yasmeen any information about the reason for my visit, so I stared at her/him startled.

Raman talked to me for over an hour. As he talked, I looked at a painting of him on the wall behind Yasmeen. In this painting there was a slight resemblance to Yasmeen, but there was no resemblance between the voice she'd used to greet me and the Middle-Eastern accented male voice I was hearing now. Yasmeen sat with her hands on her knees, occasionally gesturing to emphasise something. I asked questions and as I listened to the answers, tears gathered and began to run down my cheeks. Though Yasmeen's eyes were still closed, she paused and nodded, and Raman's voice said very softly, 'Indeed, my dear. Indeed.' She waited till I recovered myself and continued.

Raman concluded by saying that if we continued to view Rebecca's death only in terms of human life we would forever feel pain, but if we saw that her spirit hadn't died and that by being with us she'd left us a great gift, our spirituality would continue to unfold. By August I would want to rejoin the world and by the end of the year I would be ready for a big change. Going to another country would be a very positive experience for us.

At the end of the hour Raman said goodbye. Yasmeen's breathing deepened and she opened her eyes. I was so astonished at the information I'd heard that I could hardly speak except to briefly thank her. Back in my car I wept for about 20 minutes till my tears stopped and I could drive home.

Thus began my introduction to Raman. Over the following months I attended weekly sessions with him and several courses that Yasmeen ran by herself, without channelling. In one of these sessions Yasmeen described Rebecca's appearance and personality perfectly. These weekly meetings were a life raft for me and I waited impatiently for the days to pass till I could attend again.

As a language teacher I analysed Raman's vocabulary, pronunciation and grammar while replaying the cassette recordings of the sessions. However, I could find no point of similarity between the language Raman and Yasmeen used and the way they used it, nor any similarity between Yasmeen's gentle, rather shy personality and Raman's quick wit and dry humour.

At a Saturday workshop all the participants went out into the garden. Yasmeen, with her eyes closed, had no difficulty striding across the grass, or identifying each participant.

By the rose garden Yasmeen/Raman approached each person and said something which had meaning only to that individual.

Chris was scathing in his comments whenever I told him about these meetings. Finally, exasperated by his cynicism, I asked him to attend just one session with me and at least then he would know what I was talking about. If he still thought it was rubbish, I would accept that. He reluctantly agreed.

At the meeting Yasmeen passed some cards around the 20 people in the room and told us to take one and see if the picture was meaningful to the person who chose it. Chris turned his card over. It was the same picture I'd chosen myself three weeks earlier and closely resembled the painting of the vortex Rebecca had done for Burje last Christmas.

Chris looked at me and frowned. 'How odd.' He stared at his card.

As we drove home he said he was impressed with Yasmeen's gentleness and integrity. He didn't believe she was a fake. At least if she were, she herself obviously thought what she was doing was genuine. It would be hard to sustain that accent without slipping once or twice, he thought. But on the other hand, maybe she was just a good actor. It was certainly interesting that, even with her eyes closed, she/Raman knew exactly which person was asking a question. That was hard to do in a room full of people. On the other hand, there was no such thing as an afterlife. No such thing as a 3000-year-old entity being channelled through a living human being. If there were, he would have to change his whole belief system, he said, and he didn't have enough evidence to do that. So there must be a logical explanation. No, he didn't have one, but that didn't mean there wasn't one. Maybe it had something to do with multiple personality disorder. He reminded me of the charlatans we'd encountered during Rebecca's illness and that even though we were both educated, intelligent people we'd let ourselves get sucked into all that. Did I really want to go down that path again?

No, I didn't. But this felt different.

A couple of weeks after this Chris woke suddenly one night. He reached out to touch my arm.

'What are you doing *there*?'

'Where else would I be?' I muttered, cranky at being woken up.

'If you're there, who's that kneeling on the floor?'

I peered nervously over his shoulder. 'There's nobody there.'

'Yes there is. I can still see her.'

'Put the light on.'

When he did he sat up, shaken and upset. No, it wasn't Rebecca. It was a woman in her thirties. No, she wasn't scary. Very gentle, actually. However, it was obviously just a dream.

'But you were awake.'

Still, it must have been a dream, he insisted. He must have been in a sleep state, that's all. Nothing more.

He went straight back to sleep. I stayed awake the rest of the night.

Over the following years he saw coloured lights in the room, including a green and yellow patterned light over me as I lay sleeping. Occasionally he woke up to find the shape of the room had changed, or there was furniture in places that he knew were not there in daylight. These hallucinations were usually prefaced with 'Hmm. That's interesting ...' And that was how he perceived them, as interesting phenomena. During this period the sleep paralysis that had plagued him most of his life intensified and the attacks came more frequently and lasted longer. Sometimes I found it difficult to wake him from them. He consulted our GP who referred him to a sleep specialist. He had to sleep with a gadget attached to his thumb to measure his oxygen level to see whether he was suffering from sleep apnoea. Nothing untoward was found, apart from the extraordinary habit he had of dropping into REM sleep less than one minute after closing his eyes, instead of the more normal one and a half hours.

I began to dream again, but my dreams were filled with places where my children walked on surfaces that appeared to be solid, but underneath the cracked earth there was a swamp where crocodiles lay waiting. The crocodiles hid in drains, in cupboards. Just waiting. In other dreams babies died and I lost all the baby clothes I'd knitted. Rebecca played in the middle of the road and when I tried to warn her of the danger, I had no voice. Or she went missing and no one could find her then she popped up somewhere saying she'd been there all along.

Four years after Rebecca's death Chris had surgery to remove nose polyps. I read somewhere that these were caused by unshed tears. Whether or not that was true, the night-time hallucinations and sleep paralysis episodes became fewer and farther between.

As the years passed, my need for reassurance that Rebecca's life continued in some other form became less intense as I re-engaged with my own life. Nowadays, I still attend courses with Yasmeen and Raman, but less frequently, and only if I need to learn something new. The spiritual perspective I've gained from these meetings has gradually become integrated into my life. Each time I go to see Raman, it feels like going home.

# SIXTEEN

# The world turns

Two of Rebecca's friends from Art School, Jo and Christine, brought over her artwork that had remained in her studio, and a book the staff and students had made. It included photos of outings they'd been on. A couple of lecturers had written that she was one of the school's most promising, talented and successful students. A classmate had written, 'I hope she's happy, drawing and riding horses somewhere.'

They also brought us flowers and a white rose bush to plant in the garden. The mood in their class was sombre, Christine said. No one could believe it. Everyone had been on holiday when it happened, so they hadn't heard the news until they returned for the next term, fully expecting that Rebecca would be picking up from where she'd left off last September.

'Everyone used to call her Warrior Princess and Celtic Woman because she was so strong-minded and adventurous,' Jo said. When they went out onto the Port Hills to draw, Rebecca leapt from rock to rock until she fell into a gorse bush, tearing her skin. 'The blood was pouring out, but Rebecca said it didn't hurt and she carried on drawing. That's when we started the Warrior Princess thing.'

I remembered Rebecca setting out for Art School dressed in a miniskirt, riding chaps, her grandmother's green pentagram necklace, a jewel stuck between her eyebrows and studded leather bands on her wrists.

*'Omigod! You're surely not going out like that?'*

*'I'm an art student. I can dress how I like.'*

*'Hmmm ... well, I suppose that's true.'*

The girls' stories were rain in a desert. I was grateful for them and for the girls' enthusiasm about the forthcoming exhibitions that were part of their final year. When Rebecca was a first-year student I'd gone with her to one of these final-year exhibitions. She was excited as she saw the potential for her own artistic development.

I told Jo and Christine how she'd died and took them to see the horses. I told them about Fabiano and how Rebecca had found, through his actions and words, what unconditional love was. They both cried, but said they felt happy to hear the story and that hearing how she'd died helped them to accept her death.

In August we had our first social outing to the house of friends. There were 10 of us for dinner. The conversation weaved in and out of what we'd all been doing, what our children were doing, how our jobs were going, what books we'd read, what films we'd seen, how we were dealing with the aftermath of Rebecca's death, how we all viewed someone's recent suicide, the meaning of life and death. Despite the fact my composure was still only skin deep, I was able to negotiate my way around all the topics we covered. It reminded me of what normal felt like.

Next day Bart and Natasha came over. Natasha said she and her boyfriend, Daniel, had just bought a house close to Natasha's grandmother. She talked of the times she and Rebecca had gone shopping with Natasha's mother; how they'd stayed overnight at her grandmother's when they were teenagers, 'pigging out' and watching videos in their sleeping bags on the floor. When we were living in Brazil Natasha had rung Rebecca to tell her that her mother had taken her own life. I was in the kitchen at Marilena's house when Rebecca answered the phone. Her delighted shriek at the sound of Natasha's voice changed to: 'She *what*? Your *mum*?!'

She sat in a daze afterwards and talked of how much she'd liked Natasha's mum. How they'd been planning to take Rebecca to the newly opened mall in Christchurch when we returned home. How Natasha and her mother had just moved into a new flat and were enjoying themselves decorating it. When we returned to New Zealand she went with Natasha to the coroner's court.

Bart said he'd printed the photos of him and Rebecca and had them on his desk. He said he and Grant had been changed through the experience of what she'd gone through. They weren't the same any more, and her influence would always be there now and she'd always be part of their lives. As he spoke I pictured the carefree, happy young people they'd been, Grant and Bart working on their old bomb of a car in our garden, and Natasha and Rebecca showing off on the horses in the paddocks, jumping over high fences as if danger meant nothing to them and they were immortal; laughing and insulting each other in the way only people in their teens and early twenties can do, feeling beautiful and invincible.

Blair, the channeller I'd met at the death and dying seminar, was back in Christchurch and I had an appointment to see him. Just before I left the house I went into Rebecca's room and took out a green watch ring that Susannah had bought her the previous Christmas. Rebecca had adored it. I felt I wanted to have it while I was talking to Tabaash. However, it looked odd on my finger so I took it off and put it in my pocket. Then I worried I might lose it, so I put it back on the dressing table and instead wore Rebecca's half of the heart necklace she'd given to Natasha.

I had directions and a map, but I couldn't make any sense of them and kept missing the turn-off and driving into the Lyttelton Tunnel. The battery in my cellphone was flat and I arrived half an hour late and very flustered. Blair told me to take my time and calm down. There was no hurry, he said. We sat down and he immediately brought Tabaash through. Unlike Yasmeen, Blair's eyes stayed open when he channelled Tabaash. Unlike Raman, Tabaash had a very blunt way of talking and often burst into uproarious laughter. He greeted me and told me that my confusion with the map, my lack of direction and ending up in a long, dark tunnel was a metaphor for my life at present. He pointed to my hand and said, 'Where's her ring?'

My eyes widened.

'She wanted you to wear it, that's why you got the idea to go into her room and put it on.'

I explained what I'd done and he asked me to give him the necklace. As he held it in his hand he talked about aspects of Rebecca's life, her personality, her illness and dying that he couldn't possibly have known. He said Rebecca's death had enabled her to be a teacher and a healer and that hundreds of people were changed because of what had happened to her.

He told me that if I didn't start living my life and enjoying it again I'd become very ill and in so doing I would have failed Rebecca and everything she represented in her life. This blunt directive shook me, but I knew he was right.

I wrote about this visit to Sari, Susannah's friend. She responded that she'd cried when reading my letter, especially Tabaash's description of the way people's lives had been changed because of what had happened to Rebecca and she wanted to share two stories with me.

The first story began at the point where Sari had felt herself spiralling into a serious depression. Around the same time, Susannah had talked to her about Rebecca's illness and after a visit to Rebecca in hospital, Susannah had said that Rebecca just wanted to live and to spend time with her friends and get on with her life, that she hated being sick. It struck Sari that here was someone who wanted her life and didn't have a choice, while she was thinking about giving hers up. It was the story Susannah told her, she said, that made her feel thankful for her life and turned a potentially nasty depression around.

The second story centred around Susannah's request for Sari to paint a picture for her on the canvas that Rebecca had intended to use for her second painting for Susannah. Sari wrote about how honoured, but nervous, she felt about this request. She did a few preliminary sketches, playing with colour and symbols that Susannah had inspired with her stories. Most of the time the painting just flowed effortlessly, at other times she felt stuck. She'd ask Rebecca for help or would play some music and off she'd go again with a new idea. Sometimes she'd have tears streaming down her face as she repainted an area in a different tone. She was sad, but happy. Sometimes she felt the painting was getting too dark, so she lightened it up again with highlights of a different colour. She didn't know whether Rebecca helped her with the painting or not, but it involved a lot of energy and it was an amazing process for her. In that way, Rebecca touched her life again.

We finished all our work in the paddocks. It was re-fenced, the gates mended, the macrocarpa trees trimmed and the old branches cleared up and burnt, the grass fertilised and everything ready for the horses to come back in a few weeks' time, when the grass was growing well. Darryn wrote to say he would come in October to pick up Bug and Kit. He was writing a book about horsemanship and wondered if I'd help him organise and edit it.

One morning in early August I was driving to work. The sky was still dark when I set out, with a thin slice of pale moon in the sky. I thought of the frosty winter morning in England when I was around 11, leaving the house to go to school and noticing the crescent moon and a star beside it. I yelled for my mother who came running out in a panic. I pointed to the moon. 'Look! It's so beautiful!' My mother gasped in relief then tut-tutted, 'Oh, *lass*! I thought it was something important!' Now, on the other side of the world, I smiled at the memory. I remembered standing at the school bus-stop looking at the tall trees waving in the wind on the opposite side of the road and imagining what it might be like to fly like a bird over them. Over the oceans, over the mountains, to a faraway land. Now, almost half a century later, in my faraway land the sun rose over the mountains, staining the snow pink and edging the clouds with gold. I stopped the car and watched. And immediately felt guilty that I cared that the mountains looked so beautiful and the frost looked so pretty glittering on the trees. And that I liked the way mine was the only car on the road all the way to the outskirts of the city.

Winter was ending. Though there was still snow on the mountains, the first white stars of plum blossom were budding on the trees; daffodils, snowdrops, narcissi and bluebells were pushing up strong green spikes from the wet earth. The dark nights were receding, the light was returning and the days were warmer. The air smelt sweet with new grass. Lambs began filling the fields. I didn't welcome these signs of new life. I wanted to push the new green shoots back into the ground, to delay the return of the sun, to stop the cherry blossom frothing the trees, and to silence the newborn lambs. The shimmering light of spring reinforced the fact that the world had not stopped turning, and this knowledge was shocking. *This time last year she did this. This time last year we did that.*

As my birthday approached I felt only dread. On 11 September last year the collapsing towers in New York barely registered within the enormity of Rebecca's appendix bursting. This year, although I told Susannah and Benjamin I didn't want to celebrate, they both rang to say happy birthday. I felt blessed to have them. Susannah persuaded me to have my birthday dinner at her house. Reluctantly I went, with the surgeon's voice from the same-time-last-year ringing in my head.

The course I was teaching now finished. Although I'd enjoyed teaching it, I was looking forward to having a couple of weeks of quiet time. Every weekend since Rebecca's death Chris and I had been busy with work in the paddocks and gardens. Consequently, we were both now physically fit, but very tired.

I took the horses' covers off and hung them over the fence in the yard in the sun. A horse whinnied. Rebecca's voice in my head.

'*That's Red.*'

'*How do you know?*'

'*What do you mean how do I know? Don't you know which one is whinnying?*'

'*No, I don't.*'

'*But they sound completely different!*'

'*Oh.*'

Despite the fact I'd been looking forward to a rest I couldn't sit still, so I spent my two weeks' leave spring cleaning the house. While I was taking Rebecca's furniture out onto the verandah before getting the carpets shampooed, I was so overcome with sadness at picking up her things that I couldn't breathe. The last time I'd moved her things out there was a year after we'd moved into the house. We wanted to surprise her by painting her room while she was away for the weekend at an ice hockey match. Late at night we heard the familiar thunk of ice hockey skates being dropped on the verandah outside her door. She switched on the light. 'Oh. *Wow!*' She came into our room. 'It looks *great!* When did you do all *that?*'

Why did people say 'At least you have happy memories'? These were the memories that undid me. I wondered if I could sit in the garden instead, listening to the birds. This was something that used to give me great pleasure, but I'd avoided sitting still for so long that I couldn't stop springing out of my seat. So the garden was filled with birdsong? So what? Back to the cleaning.

Susannah said she hadn't really let her grief out when Rebecca died because she couldn't believe it or accept it and the physical pain was intense. 'I can't cry,' she said. 'The tears are all inside. It feels like bleeding inside.'

Benjamin began talking about Rebecca, which he'd avoided doing since she died. He said he was missing her and being in Wellington made her death seem unreal. He was thinking of returning to Christchurch to live after he had some more experience in his present job. He felt the time in Wellington had been wasted when he could have been with Rebecca. Anger characterised his grief. He said he felt like kicking rubbish bins and letter boxes as he walked to work. He sat on the roof alone in his lunch hour and ate his sandwiches there. He didn't want to talk to people. He'd made no friends in Wellington and didn't want any. If he'd had the choice of saving his sister or saving a country he would have let the country be destroyed, he said.

There was a Festival of Dance on in the city. It was the first time Chris and I had been out together for dinner and a show for almost two years. We bumped into two friends and had coffee with them afterwards in a wine bar that had live music. We also had tickets for another two shows that week. The third one was a solo dance performance of astonishing grace. We were both amazed that something of beauty still existed that had the power to move us to such a degree.

At the end of the month a Cuban dance show came to Christchurch so we bought tickets for that too. *Lady Salsa* was a visual history of the development of Cuban music and was full of energy and exuberance. It reminded us of Brazil. In the interval we met Gail and Paulo. I'd met Gail at the Portuguese classes we'd attended on our return from Brazil. I'd given them a package to give to Fabiano when they went to Brazil on business and they'd liked him enormously and had kept in touch with him. He'd told Gail of his sadness when Rebecca rejected him and he'd told her of his despair when he'd seen her dying. Paulo had lived in New Zealand for so long that when he went back to Brazil his family told him he didn't walk like a Brazilian any more. The friend who was with them said, 'You mean there's a Kiwi walk?' It was very funny and we laughed. The sound of our laughter felt strange and unfamiliar.

In September we were in the garden when, above the noise of the nor'west wind, I heard the phone ring. It was Chris's colleague, Jos, who'd been instrumental in persuading us to come to New Zealand 26 years before. They'd both worked at Manchester University in England and when Jos was offered a chair in Electrical Engineering at Canterbury he persuaded Chris to join the team when he'd completed his PhD. They had four children. The third one, Elizabeth, was in England on her OE.

It took me a moment to realise he wasn't laughing. He was crying. 'Elizabeth is dead,' he sobbed.

She'd been knocked off her bike by a taxi in the middle of London. She hadn't been wearing a helmet.

After I put the phone down Chris and I sat with our heads in our hands, the sunshine all gone out of the day.

Elizabeth's funeral in the local Catholic church was much bigger and more formal than Rebecca's little gathering of close friends in our garden. I observed the sorrow of her friends as they spoke about her. The music. The sprinkling of soil on her coffin. The colleagues and friends giving support, but grieving too. I regretted that we hadn't invited more people to farewell Rebecca. I asked Chris if he thought we were wrong to exclude so many people. No, he said. Rebecca hated fuss and formality.

Darryn wrote to say he'd pick Bug and Kit up at the end of October. Kit's summer coat had come in and she was a lovely dark chestnut with a gorgeous orange mane and tail. She looked stunning. Rebecca would have been delighted with the way she was growing up. Bug had lost some of his excess fat in the winter and was trotting and cantering around the paddocks with much more energy. I thought of the rapport Rebecca had with him. When she'd taken him on a trek two years earlier she'd ridden him bareback for six hours. People still told me how they'd seen her galloping bareback on Bug up a steep hill, with just a halter on him. I was so glad we'd had this beautiful, gentle animal in our lives for three years. I stroked his nose.

Rebecca's voice: '*Wow!* I can't *believe* it! I've got a *quarterhorse!*'

She'd be happy for him and Kit to go to Darryn. I couldn't wish for a better home for them.

An hour or so before Darryn arrived I sat in the paddock and bawled my eyes out. However, when he loaded them onto his truck I knew that the time was right for them to go. He was keeping Bug to ride on his cattle station in Alexandra and cutting cattle was exactly what Bug was bred for. Nicky, Darryn's wife was very excited at the thought of having Bug back again. She'd also fallen in love with Kit. Darryn would start training Kit and if he decided not to keep her he would find her a good home. He asked me to go into the truck and rub their noses to say goodbye. Red and Jade, still in the paddock, ran around snorting indignantly at the departure of their friends.

Benjamin's 28th and Susannah's 32nd birthdays were in October and we had a combined celebration for them. I bought Benjamin some clothes for his birthday, including a pair of baggy shorts that Susannah had assured me were very trendy. When he took them out of the packet they looked enormous.

'What? D'ya think I've turned into Fatty Arbuckle?' He laughed so hard he couldn't breathe and tears flooded his cheeks. Chris started laughing too and that started the rest of us off. I realised it was the first time for at least a year that we'd laughed like that. Benjamin's laughter was exactly like Rebecca's, full-bodied and bubbling. They'd shared the same sense of humour as Chris and the same gasping-for-breath, tears-pouring-down-the-cheeks, bent-over-helpless, stomach-clutching way of laughing. As I watched Chris and Benjamin rolling around in their chairs, I couldn't remember the last time I'd heard either of them laugh like that. Susannah looked at me and smiled.

Rebecca had worked so hard to get in to the Art and Design course and we had looked forward to seeing her graduate. Her friends would soon be graduating. Their final exhibition was being held at the CoCA Gallery and Chris and I had an invitation to go.

We looked at the work on display and read the names of the artists we'd heard

Rebecca talking about so often. Jo had always painted fairies, she said. But in her powerfully depicted feminist images there was no trace now of a fairy. Christine saw us and told us how she couldn't believe the course was ending. The three years had been filled with incredibly hard work, but lots of fun, she said. Rebecca was acknowledged in the catalogue along with the fact she'd 'lost her battle with cancer'. I wondered where her work would have been displayed. I wondered what it would have been like.

It was the end of my lesson and I was hurrying along the corridor of level two, looking forward to getting a cup of coffee. Below, a group of students stood chatting in the atrium. With a shock I noted that one girl was the same height and body shape as Rebecca. Her long, fair hair was tied back in a ponytail. She was even standing in the same posture as Rebecca had, reading something she was holding in one hand and nibbling the nails of her other hand. This was the first time I'd seen anyone who resembled Rebecca at all. I stood watching her for a few minutes.

Three years after this incident I was working in my study one dark evening when there was a tap on my window. I peered into the dark porch to see who it was. With a shock I saw Rebecca. My first thought was 'She's come back.' It was at the level of consciousness that accompanies the first second of waking in the morning. As full remembrance dawned on me, I saw the person was not Rebecca. It was my neighbour, probably wondering why I was gawking at her like that. I opened the front door with knees shaking and invited her in. I decided to say nothing. I didn't want to sound unhinged.

Two years later I saw a teenage girl on a ferry on the way back from Great Keppel Island in Australia. She had the same hair colour, skin tone and facial expression as Rebecca. I watched her as subtly as I could and would have taken a photograph if I hadn't thought it would look extremely odd.

As we got off the boat Susannah said, 'Mum! Did you see that girl?'

I nodded.

'Oh, she looked so like Rebecca. I couldn't believe it!'

'Yes, she did.'

She asked Chris if he'd noticed the girl. No, he hadn't.

The academic year was finished. Summer holidays and Christmas were approaching. Benjamin and Dee and Elliot would stay with us for three weeks. I had no interest in celebrating Christmas. Rebecca had loved this season and she and Chris had always decorated the tree together after we moved to Greendale. I decided not to get a tree, nor bring down the ornaments from the attic. We'd have a simple family dinner and exchange presents. This-time-last-year was no longer something I wished to remember. The photographs we'd taken the previous Christmas showed Rebecca getting thinner and thinner. Benjamin told me it was at that time he knew Rebecca wouldn't recover.

'I knew it. Dad knew it. Susannah knew it. You were the only one who wouldn't accept it, Mum,' he said.

'It wasn't a case of not accepting it,' I said. 'I didn't know.'

I looked at her clothes in her cupboard and all her things on her desk. I felt I would drown in my own tears.

In the summer holidays a trainer who'd studied with Pat Parelli in the USA came out to help me with Jade. I was looking forward to doing some walking and swimming. But I couldn't lie in the hammock and read. I couldn't sit still. I couldn't plan the future. I couldn't think about the past. The empty spaces were still full of empty.

# Time to leave again

After the New Year our friend Helen arrived from the USA on a visit. Her last visit had been two years before, when Helen's father had died and she'd brought her mother to Greendale. Rebecca had shown them around the garden and paddocks before dashing off to an ice hockey game. Now, on this visit, they came to comfort us. I admired Helen enormously for her determination to become a kidney specialist, to be a partner in her own clinic, and to sustain a long and happy marriage through the years of separation that medical school had brought. Above all I loved her enthusiasm for life and her sense of humour. Chris said she was the most down-to-earth, most high-achieving, yet modest person he'd ever met.

Before they left, we showed them Rebecca's paintings, which we'd had framed. One was of her Siamese cat, Sing, poised to kill. In the reflection of the cat's blue eyes stood a tiny mouse, hands on hips, mocking the idea of death.

After they returned home to Texas, Helen emailed me. She said that as she was driving from our house she heard Rebecca's voice saying she wanted to be with me, but was unable to because of my pain and that she'd wanted to die like a child. Helen thought this had something to do with the way she faced death, as if it came from behind while she looked forward.

*Several times I have received messages like this that are unexplainable, but very calm and clear. I wonder if it is because I work constantly with death. I really have no explanation. I keep thinking about the message in the cat's eyes. What a great way to see life!*

I asked her to elaborate and she wrote that she felt that Rebecca had been waiting for her to give me the message and that there was a sense of urgency about it.

*I remember the phrase 'I am there' (in your home). She finds it hard to be there because she is seeking tranquility and 'I want to be in her' (I knew it meant you) 'but I need peace to be there (in you) and there is too much pain and busyness.' I think it is time now you processed the pain so you can give her the peace she needs and I think the healing will begin soon. It is as if she is giving you permission to feel less pain and celebrate her life.*

*I think you will naturally slow down soon. She was not ready to die as she enjoyed life and there were still things she wanted to do but her body gave out. Rather than having to process death she chose to die as a child by going to sleep with her family around her. It was easier for her and she was weary. One other thing she said was 'you saw my art'. There was playfulness in the message. I think there are so many messages in the art that will make you smile – like the big pointy ears on the faces. You need to talk to her as she wants to be part of your life.*

Chris was shaken by Helen's messages. He had the greatest respect for her intelligence and integrity and therefore couldn't dismiss her as a crank as he so readily did others.

'Perhaps that was why Rebecca chose her,' I suggested.

He shrugged. He didn't know. He just didn't know.

For Chris's 60th birthday we took him for a surprise dinner on the restaurant tram in Christchurch. As it circled around the city Mark talked about movies he and Susannah had seen. Rebecca would've loved them, he said. Rebecca would've loved this music and that music. Did I remember when she said …? Wasn't it funny the way she …? He cried when he spoke about her, but I was immensely grateful for the way he spoke her name, as though it were the most natural thing in the world.

One day when Rebecca was in hospital we noticed she was lying with her toes clamped around the bar of the bed. As each visitor came in Susannah asked Rebecca to demonstrate her double joints. By the time Mark came in Rebecca was fed up with being asked to do this and said no. Mark said, 'Rebecca, you said you love me like a brother. Well, I won't believe you unless you curl your toes around the bar.'

Rebecca burst out laughing and obliged with a demonstration.

Before she got cancer he'd taken her out on his father's motorbike. He'd swum with her in the pool at home. He'd thrown her into the water. He'd made her laugh till she doubled over. He'd lifted her into her coffin and helped carry the coffin to the hearse. He was one of the few who mentioned her name now.

Darryn was back in Darfield running a horsemanship clinic over four days. I couldn't ride because my foot was in plaster from minor surgery, so Sue rode Jade in my place while I watched with my foot wrapped up in a plastic bag. The last time I'd been in this place was with Rebecca, 17 months ago. With the first anniversary of her death looming the following weekend, four days at the horse clinic was a good place to be.

When Sue loaded Jade into the horse float for the first time in 17 months we expected he'd resist, but he just strolled in. She told Darryn that she'd done it the way Rebecca had shown her, which was the way Rebecca had learned it from him. He smiled a big, slow smile.

Some of the participants remembered Rebecca from previous clinics and lessons. One young woman asked where she was. How come she wasn't at the clinic? Had she finished her degree? Was she travelling overseas now? I told her Rebecca had died a year ago. The girl stared at me and her eyes filled with tears. Her mother had died of cancer two years before. She knew what that was like, she said. She told me about a trek on the beach the riding group had been on. The wheel on her horse float had broken. Rebecca helped her fix it and lent her some tools.

'She was the first person to welcome me on that trek,' she said. 'She was so chatty and friendly. Did she know then …?'

'Yes, she did.'

Another woman remembered Rebecca riding our big old Clydesdale bareback three years ago, at one of the clinics. Everybody had been amazed to see her do it, she said. Rebecca had always been the first to come up and speak to her and welcome her to the riding club. Another woman told me she used to work in the oncology ward and although she hadn't met Rebecca because she was on leave at the time, she said she knew all about her.

To hear other people speak her name and tell me her stories was the most beautiful gift they could have given me.

The first anniversary. I opened the front door and in flew a fantail. We wept.

Later that morning we went to Hanmer Springs for the day. The little alpine village had been a favourite when the children were young. We walked up a steep track through the bush and said to each other, 'Remember when ...?' Back home we lit a candle and between 9.15 and 10.15pm we sat silently in the candlelight. We placed a rose on Rebecca's bed.

All week rain drenched the land. The farmers, frantic about the drought, welcomed the deluge that would transform the barren desert the Canterbury Plains had become to lush green pastures.

Having my foot in plaster was a good excuse to withdraw from the world. I'd avoided going onto the verandah since we'd put Rebecca's coffin there. Every time I walked near the area I thought of her cats sitting by her coffin and Elliot dancing in front of it in time to the music. After the fantail's visit, I went out onto the verandah and allowed myself to remember. Rebecca drawing and painting with her cats and ferrets running beside her; Rebecca playing with the dogs; feeding the newborn goat she'd brought home and laughing when I mistook it for a sheepskin slipper; sleeping on the verandah with Natasha when they aborted their attempt to camp in the paddock next to the horses after they'd seen something unexplainable in the sky and got spooked; sleeping on the verandah with Natasha and Fabiano under the full moon while he sang opera arias to them on his first visit here; Grant and Bart sleeping on the verandah, with Natasha and Rebecca hurling insults at them through the open bedroom window, telling jokes and roaring with laughter while Chris and I requested that they please turn the volume down a bit so we could get some sleep; Rebecca and I sitting on the verandah while she told me that when she had children she wouldn't pamper them. She'd have them in the saddle with her from the first week. They'd run around the garden naked and feel the sun on their skin.

'Oh, so your poor little six-month-old will be crawling around on the grass in the rain with no clothes on?'

'Oh well, okay, I'll put a vest on him.'

'Him?'

'Yeah. I want a couple of boys. You can do more with them than girls. Sports and riding and stuff.'

'*You* haven't done too badly.'

'Well, maybe a boy and a girl then.'

'If you have a girl I'll buy her pink dresses!'

'Hmmmmm!'

'Not that it worked with you though, did it?'

I allowed these thoughts to drift. Sue came over and sat with me. She'd been in the horse paddock the previous night, she said, just sitting there watching the full moon rise from behind a cloud.

Rebecca's birthday on 9 May was approaching. Susannah dreamt that Rebecca was helping to prepare for her birthday and she asked Susannah if she'd bought any presents. In the dream Susannah was aware that Rebecca was no longer living and didn't know how to reply. Rebecca then told her to buy a present for Elliot.

On 9 May the skies were blue, the air warm, the leaves on the pin oak turning crimson. It was the same kind of balmy autumn weather as the day Rebecca was born and the day she died. We had a family dinner and burned a candle all day. Chris loaded photographs of Rebecca from the computer on to his digital camera and then offloaded them on to the television screen. There were photographs from her newborn days to just before she got sick. The photos made us cry, but we also laughed and they triggered stories of 'Remember when she ...?'

The next day we went to Willowbank, the wildlife reserve. The last time we'd been there was the day Fabiano declared his love for Rebecca, five years earlier. Willowbank had been one of her favourite places when she was growing up. Elliot, now two and a half, loved the animals and birds. I showed him a beautiful, bright green parrot and when we walked away from it he said, 'Bye. Bye. Lovely. Green. Bird.' We all laughed. I realised I still didn't laugh very often, but when I did, I no longer felt guilty.

We planned on leaving New Zealand on 21 June and travelling to England to spend a week with my brother and visit some friends. We would arrive in Oman on 3 July and I'd begin teaching there on 7 July. When I'd finished my year-long contract, we'd fly to Brazil for a few days and then on to Washington to visit Marilena, who was now living there with her new husband, Bernard. We had to be back in New Zealand by 20 June 2004, according to the terms of our 12-month ticket. Susannah wept. 'A whole year without you.'

'But you understand, don't you?'

She did.

# EIGHTEEN

# Connecting with the past

At Newcastle Airport my brother Tom strode towards us. I almost fell into his arms. Chris and I hadn't been back to England together for 22 years, when Susannah was 11, Benjamin seven and Rebecca three.

'You've turned into Dad!' I said, hugging him tight.

'Watch it or I'll say you've turned into Mam!' he laughed, wrapping me in a bear hug.

When we arrived at his house, his wife, Val, was waiting for us and we met their two children, Paul, aged 15 and Laura, aged 13, for the first time. Tom had sent me a photo of Laura a few months earlier and when I'd first seen the photo of the slim, blonde girl with golden arms and legs my breath caught in my throat. She could have been Rebecca at the same age. To test that this wasn't just my imagination I showed the photo to Chris, Susannah and Benjamin, Grant, Bart and Natasha. They all assumed it was Rebecca. I'd been looking forward to meeting her with some trepidation. I wanted so much for her to look exactly like Rebecca in the flesh, but as she came into the kitchen I could see she didn't.

'What do you think?' asked Tom.

I shook my head. 'There's a resemblance, but it must've been just the way you captured her for that photo.'

He told me that when Rebecca became ill Laura had found some photos of the cousin she'd never met and arranged them in little frames in her room. After my initial disappointment that Laura was not a Rebecca clone, I was able to enjoy getting to know the girl she really was. Laura was very feminine and loved clothes. That was one of the major differences between her and Rebecca. When we went out one evening with friends of Tom and Val, one of them said she was astonished at the resemblance of Laura to me. As Rebecca and I looked alike, her comment pleased me very much. Paul, at 15, was already taller than his father, and very shy and sweet. I wondered why it had taken me so long to come and see them. Where had all the years gone?

That night as we sat in their living room Val asked hesitantly, 'Sandra … can I ask? … how was it?'

We let our tears flow freely as we talked about how it was.

Living with them in that week was like sinking into an old, warm, familiar bean bag. I was enclosed, embraced, cosseted. We caught up on all the missing years, watched videos of their children growing up, showed them our own family photos. When they saw the video Sebastião had taken of us in Brazil they laughed at a shot of Rebecca rolling her eyes in annoyance at something. 'Now *that's* Laura's expression to a T!' Tom hooted.

Paul and Laura were curious about our life in New Zealand and also about the life Tom and I had when we were growing up.

'Did you fight much?' asked Laura.

'No, not much,' Tom and I said simultaneously.

And my brother and I began to retrace the steps of our childhood.

First we went to Washington where we'd grown up. We drove past our old home where little had changed except there was a car parked in what had been our mother's garden. The last time we'd been there Rebecca was three and a half and my family hadn't yet met her. My mother was waiting at the back door to scoop this new granddaughter into her arms and hug her tight, before she wrapped her arms around all of us. When we left for New Zealand again eight months later my mother's tears were for her conviction that she wouldn't see us again. She died less than a year later.

At the cemetery we put flowers on the graves of our parents and grandparents and walked around the church where Chris and I were married. We visited an old family friend, Mabel, who was now 80. She'd been 60 on my last brief visit and she'd comforted me over the death of my mother, explaining to me in detail what had happened, how both my parents knew my mother had cancer. How neither of them would admit it to the other. How she'd urged my father to write and tell me, but he'd left it too late because that would have meant admitting to himself that she was going to die. Now, she could summon no words to comfort me over the death of my child. She drew on her religion. 'Always remember pet, God never sends us more than we can bear.'

She meant it kindly and I thanked her.

I told her I always remembered her as extremely glamorous, especially when she and her husband and my parents went to the Masonic dances at Christmas. Her fabulous dresses, filled with sequins, her sparkling jewellery, fur coat and gorgeous perfumes. As a child I'd always looked forward to the sight. I'd thought she looked like a princess, I said.

She smiled. 'Ah, pet, that was a long time ago.'

An email from Joan in Oman informed me that Abdul, the CEO, said my visa still wasn't ready and asked me to postpone our flight to Oman for a week. That suited me because now we'd have a week longer in England, but warning lights were starting to flash about the wisdom of our choice in going to Oman. My gut feeling had told me not to leave New Zealand without the visa.

When Rebecca was first diagnosed with cancer Tom had spoken to her on the phone and asked her to paint him a self-portrait. She'd started a sketch of herself in a cowboy hat, but hadn't liked it enough to continue with it. Before we left New Zealand we searched through her paintings and found one she'd done of herself as a four-year-old child blowing a dandelion clock. It was taken from a photograph where she was wearing a jersey knitted by my mother on our last trip to England. We framed the painting and Tom hung it on his living room wall. We took a photo of Laura standing beside it. I was glad to know that some of Rebecca's art was now here in England with this branch of her family.

Tom got out a box of photos that he'd retrieved from our father's house after he died. Some of them I hadn't seen before. Especially poignant were three postcards from our father to his mother and one from her to him on his 15th birthday. He'd told us many stories about his childhood, playing football in the streets, refusing his parents' commands to practise the piano till, exasperated, they let him out to get back to his football. However, we hadn't known the address of his old home before, so we decided to go and see if the house still existed.

We located the house in Wallsend where he'd grown up. *This is where he played football*, I thought, *here in these narrow, grey streets*. I had no photographs of him as a child and I tried to picture him inside this house, sitting in front of a piano he refused to play. We found the house where he'd lived with his sister who'd looked after him when their parents died. She was six years older and a brilliant pianist, he'd said many times. When he was 21 she'd died suddenly of peritonitis, leaving behind a husband and two-year-old daughter. My father was so devastated by her death he left home and joined the Merchant

Navy and never went back. Thus, the loss of all his photographs. We stood staring at the house, trying to remember whether our father, whose name was also Tom, had been 17 or 21 when his sister had bought him a motorbike. I thought 17. My brother was sure the bike had been his 21st birthday present. Val suddenly whispered, 'Omigod!' and pointed to a car parked outside the house. The registration plate declared in bold, black letters: **W TOM 21**.

We all looked at each other, the hairs on our necks standing up.

From Oman came the news that the visa would be delayed even longer as they now needed to have our marriage certificate verified. It seemed that Omani bureaucracy was in a class of its own. When I told my brother we'd paid for our own return air tickets and the company would refund mine when we arrived in Oman, the accountant in him sucked in his breath.

'Are you sure?'

'Oh yes, it's in the contract.'

'Is the contract signed?'

'Not yet.'

He raised his eyebrows.

We used the extra time to visit friends and familiar places. The immersion into ancient history revitalised my spirit. I realised how much I'd missed that since living in New Zealand. In a museum on Hadrian's Wall we looked at leather, studded wristbands that were very like the ones Rebecca had made for herself when she was working on an assignment about Roman architecture. 'She'd have loved all this,' was our constant refrain.

In a country pub we met up with Arline, an old friend from student days. Our conversation began as if we'd never left off 20 years earlier. We talked about the night she travelled by train to London, soon after we'd graduated, expecting that another friend, Sue, would get on the train at York. They were going to France together for a holiday. Most of us had had our 21st parties by then, but Sue, resisting all our efforts at persuasion, said she wasn't going to have one. On our last night at college, as we all talked about our future plans, Sue said she intended to study Spanish then go to South America to teach English. I looked at her and had an impression of darkness around her that was so strong I had to leave the room. My friend Marj followed me and asked what was wrong.

'I couldn't see a future for Sue,' I said.

'Well, that's probably just because we're all sad at the thought of leaving each other after three years.'

'Probably.'

Sue didn't get on the train at York so Arline waited at the station in London for the next train to arrive. A policeman approached her. He was sorry to tell her that Sue had been killed with both her parents on the way to York station.

Marj rang my mother and told her the news and also what I'd said about Sue having no future. My mother broke the news to me at home.

'What you thought – about Sue – it doesn't mean anything,' she assured. 'It was just a coincidence. And *please* don't mention it to your auntie.'

My mother had no patience with her sister's involvement in spiritualism.

None of us could believe the news.

Even at the funeral.

Even when we saw the three coffins at the front of the church.

Even when Sue's grandmother almost fainted in the front pew.

Not even when two friends said they had gone to see Sue's body.

Not even then.


'I still think of her every day,' said Arline. 'I can't imagine what it must be like for you. With Rebecca.'


At the end of three weeks we said goodbye to my brother and his family.

'You've put a smile back on my face,' I told Tom, not wanting to let him go so soon.

'Don't leave it so long before your next visit,' he said, fighting back his own tears.

I promised we wouldn't.

In a little village outside Henley, we stayed with our friends Marj and Alfie. Their home was the old school house with the 200-year-old school next door. They'd been in the house for two years and had renovated it beautifully with soft, quiet colours, books lining the walls, and a grand piano. They'd had a request from the BBC for permission to film an episode of *Midsomer Murders* there. Alfie had given us a pen-and-ink drawing of Alnwick Castle that he'd done as a parting gift when we'd left for the USA in 1970. Now, as an advisor for the Department of Education, he had no time for painting, he said sadly.

The windows of the house overlooked the old village church, and young girls rode their horses in the lane past the garden gate. The garden was full of flowers and climbing roses; robins sang in the vine over the hand pump by the well. Bethan, their daughter, was 21, no longer the baby I remembered, and was studying psychology at Warwick University. Rebecca, who was 24, was working in London. When Marj and I gave birth to girls, we discovered we'd both chosen the name Rebecca. As I was in New Zealand and she was in England we decided it wouldn't cause any confusion.

In the British Museum in London we headed straight for the Lindow Man exhibition. I'd waited 15 years to see it, since I'd bought the book *The Life and Death of a Druid Prince* for Rebecca, written by one of the archaeologists who'd excavated the site in Cheshire in 1984. There was an artist's reconstruction of what he'd probably looked like.

'Oh, how she would have loved all this!'

On our last night in England we sat in a village pub with Marj and Alfie, Bethan and her boyfriend. A full moon hung over the trees and the scent of honeysuckle was thick in the summer air. So much to talk about, so little time to catch up.

We talked about the musical Alfie had organised for schools in the district, Marj's work in special education, Bethan's plans after university, Rebecca's life in London and her thoughts of postgraduate work. I liked hearing Marj say 'Rebecca', even though it was not my Rebecca we were talking about. I tried to bring her into the conversation a few times, but my words just hung in the air with nowhere to go.

We waved goodbye to Marj and Alfie, still talking as we drove away, promising not to wait another 20 years, and headed to Heathrow. That night we would fly to Dubai. I saw some men in white Arab robes and headdresses in the airport and with a thrill of anticipation I thought, *We're going to the Middle East!*

Many months later Marj wrote and explained that she didn't talk about Rebecca in case it caused us pain. It took me many more months before I could articulate that not talking about Rebecca caused me much *more* pain.

# NINETEEN

# A year in Oman

Driving through Muscat was like travelling through the *Arabian Nights* of my childhood imagination, yet the city, surrounded by jagged, toffee-coloured mountains, had sprouted from the desert in only 30 years. Traditional Arabian architecture with arched windows and doors in soft shades of pink, sand and cream lined the flower-filled streets in the new part of the city. Mosques with blue and gold minarets, palaces, forts and old white-latticed Portuguese houses filled the old part. Long stretches of golden beach fringed the clear, turquoise sea in which whole families swam together, the women fully dressed in their saris or abayas. I supposed the sun was hot enough to dry their clothes while they stood on the beach.

Enormous roundabouts, profusely decorated with native trees and flowers, were further embellished by artist-commissioned sculptures. These took the form of an incense burner, a coffee pot and cups, fish, a dhow, and a fort complete with canons. Each day armies of Indians swooped on the roads with their brooms. Coloured lights illuminated some of the rock formations lining the roads into the city; others were painted with murals, or decorated with mosaics or artificial waterfalls. The scent of frankincense and frangipani permeated the air. I was glad we'd made the decision to come here. I saw in this magical place possibilities for our recovery.

It's Christmas Eve and we're sailing in the Gulf of Oman. Past empty beaches, yachts, a couple of wooden dhows. The tide is out when we arrive at the bay. The two Omani crew members and Talin, our guide, carry all the camping equipment to the beach then the

Omanis board the boat again, leaving Talin and us behind. I'm grateful they don't call out Merry Christmas.

While Talin sets up the tents, Chris and I explore. Mountains the colour of caramel rise behind the white sand and clear blue sea. From the top of a rock we see pinpricks of light from the blue and gold minarets, the palaces and forts, the old, white-latticed houses by the harbour, the market crammed with black-clad women and white-robed men, the clamour of voices, and the drift of frankincense. But from that place to this lies a long curve of empty beach, an empty sky and an empty sea. We might be the only people on earth.

Not quite.

There's Talin on the beach below, stacking driftwood in violet light. Within minutes he's wrapped in darkness. He sets a match to the fire and is silhouetted like a shadow-puppet in flames. As we clamber down the rock, a couple of fishing boats arrive. The fishermen wave, call to Talin, set their nets and take off again, swallowed by the night. The wake of their boat agitates the algae, setting off sparks of luminescence that edge each wave with silver. Chris grabs my hand and pulls me laughing into the sea. Our bodies are coated with tiny silver stars. We swim in stars until Talin calls out that our meal is ready.

As we eat by the fire, Talin tells us he's been doing this job for 10 years. He sends money back to his family in Pakistan, and visits them every two years on his one month vacation. After his last vacation his wife became pregnant with their fourth child, his first son, whom he hasn't yet seen. Chris says it must be difficult being separated from his family and not seeing his baby son.

He doesn't answer.

The air is so hot we leave the tent open all night and sleep in the light of a new moon. I dream of paper lanterns and magic castles and sliding down a snow-covered hill. I dream of kaleidoscopes and crayons and church bells and fairy tales. And dolls' prams and chocolate coins and oranges in stockings by the chimney. I dream of my friend, Sue, killed in a car crash at 20. I tell her she still looks young while we've all grown old. I take her hand and feel her soft, cool skin. I say it's terrible that she died so young. She shrugs, and says at the moment of dying the perspective is different, and you realise nothing has changed, and your life continues just the same. I argue that I can't see how not having a body is better. She says what you lack in space is made up for by other things.

The dream shakes me awake. I want to slide back to kaleidoscopes and spinning tops. The sleigh and the snowman. It's the hour when babies slip into the world and old people slip out of it, and sometimes those in between. Chris murmurs, deep inside dreams of his own. I slip outside the tent. The sky is packed with stars. Fat blobs of light. I reach up to see if I can touch them. *Rebecca, at seven, stretching up to the top of the Christmas tree with her cut-out star.*

I walk into the waves with my baby in my arms and set her adrift on the sea. A bird flies low overhead.

When I wake again, the blackness of night has drained out of the rocks and sand leaving them pale and insipid. I want to tell Chris about my dreams, but he is already in the sea. Talin is boiling water on the fire for coffee. The fishermen return to collect their nets. They wave and sail away as sunlight stains the peaks with gold.

*Rebecca at 10, bringing me her cardboard mountains with a strip of orange tissue paper behind to make the sunrise glow. Rebecca at 20, working on Kevin's farm in Hororata. 'It was foggy and I couldn't see the mountains. When the fog cleared and the Alps were visible I knew I was home.'*

Crabs run about digging frantically, the males leaving towers of sand to attract females. Tiny pink shells glitter like rubies. The sea is a mirror of the sky. I run in and shatter clouds. We've sent no cards this Christmas, bought no presents, stuffed no stockings with oranges. But the sun rolls over the mountains like a giant orange, painting the sea with light.

Talin waves to let us know he has breakfast ready and waiting – fresh croissants, hot coffee and mince pies.

'Merry Christmas!' he shouts, looking pleased with himself.

They're just words, we tell each other. They're not kaleidoscopes, or paintboxes, or roller skates. They're not Christmas trees with a cut-out star on top. They're not saddles gathering dust in the barn. They're not ashes in the earth under a rowan tree. What they are is a man far from home. And purple shadows on a sandy beach. And crackling flames in a driftwood fire. And silver stars in an inky sea. And fishermen waving on a blue and gold morning.

Talin smiles from ear to ear.

We swim to the shore and tell each other our dreams.

Such dreams.

Oh such dreams.

Darryn wrote to say Bug had died. His arthritis was so bad that Darryn had euthanised him and buried him under the tree where he loved to stand.

I wept.

'All three of her favourite horses are with her,' said Chris. 'Cristiane, Beija-Flor, and now Bug.'

On 5 April Chris and I drove over steep winding roads, past mangrove swamps and lagoons to As Seefar Beach, where the mountains rose behind a long, curved, white-sand bay and clear, green sea. We wanted to spend the second anniversary of Rebecca's death alone. After setting up camp on a dune, we ate our evening meal as the sun dropped behind the horizon and light drained from the day. We left the tent flap open all night and fell asleep watching the reflection of the moon on the sea, and fluorescent sparks dancing off the waves.

In the morning we were up early to watch the sun pour colour into the pale grey of early dawn. After breakfast we went for a swim and a long walk, frequently dipping back into the sea to cool off. Soon, the sun was blazing. We knelt in the sea with the water up to our shoulders and started talking about Rebecca and the night she died. This was the first time we'd been able to discuss that night and articulate the feelings of desolation that sat like rocks in the centre of our chests.

Seagulls keened. The long stretches of empty beach. Empty sky. Empty ocean. Chris suddenly reached down into the sea and brought up a stone. He looked at it for a long time and held it out to me, in silence. I glanced at the flat, grey, oval stone covered in limpets.

'What?'

'Look at it! Can't you see?' He had tears in his eyes.

I looked closely. In the middle of the stone was a pattern of white calcification where the limpets had dropped off. The pattern formed a perfectly shaped R. It was etched in the same design, with the same curls on the down strokes as the R Rebecca had chosen for her key ring on her last Christmas, the day we'd gone shopping for red paper to background the horse she'd painted for Elliot.

Later, sitting on the sand, staring at the stone, we had no words to explain away what we were looking at. Finally, Chris reached for his watch.

'I found it at two o'clock,' he said.

I nodded, tracing the outline of the R with my fingertip.

'Two o'clock here was ten o'clock at night in New Zealand,' he said.

I leaned against him. 'The time she died.'

Oman gave us a year of adventure in a magical landscape. I soothed my soul with visits to ancient archaeological sites, relaxed my body with long, leisurely swims in the warm, turquoise sea, reawakened my senses in the kaleidoscopic colours and exotic sounds and scents of the markets. I rediscovered my sense of humour with colleagues who made me laugh so much it hurt. Oman gave me students I'll always remember for their curiosity and willingness to learn, their sweetness, their humour and their grace; students who helped me remember how much I loved teaching. It also gave us frustrating bureaucracy and employers who were well practised in dodging their contractual obligations and who flicked off every request with 'No problem, I'll get back to you on this, *inshallah* (if God wills)'. It gave me back, in the end, the mental acuity I needed to stay one step ahead of them. All this is another story.

Except …

In the office the accountant showed me a book of blank cheques and smiled. He was very sorry, but he'd be unable to pay me my last month's salary with holiday pay and gratuities. He would, however, send a driver to the town where the sheik was staying and get him to sign a cheque. If the sheik could be found the money might be in my account on Thursday. Or Saturday. Or Sunday. Anyway, sometime soon. Failing that, they'd send it to me in New Zealand. He'd get back to me, *inshallah*.

As my brother had predicted, I'd lost the battle to get the company to refund my return airfare, so I wasn't about to leave Oman without my salary safely in the bank.

'So why can't you just give it to me in cash?'

'Unfortunately, I don't have the cash.'

'You're saying that despite this company owning hotels and travel agencies, you don't have enough cash to pay me.'

'Correct.'

In that case, I said, Chris would fly to Brazil alone next week. Regrettably, I'd miss our friend's wedding there, but I'd stay in Oman by myself till all the money was in the bank. Until it was, I'd withhold my end-of-course reports to the Ministry of Higher Education, which had sponsored my students and I'd send an email to my students and the ministry to explain why.

The accountant's smirk frayed a little around the edges as he weighed up the odds that I was bluffing. The manager's sharp intake of breath convinced him otherwise. He picked up the phone and asked for the cash to be brought over that evening.

'It will be in your account in the morning, *inshallah*.'

'Excellent.'

He could barely contain his annoyance. 'When you leave Oman next week the PRO will accompany you to the airport to cancel your visa. There you will return your Labour Card to him.'

'Of course.'

'And your Alcohol Licence.'

'Naturally.'

'And you'll need to teach the evening classes this week.'

'No problem.'

'So when are you actually leaving? Ahmed will need to inspect your flat.'

'Because …?'

'Because you might have broken something.' His composure was returning now.

'I'll check the date and time of the flight and let you know,' I purred.

Next morning, 10 minutes before the bank was due to close for the weekend, I watched the accountant hand over my salary to the teller – minus the return airfare. I transferred the money to New Zealand while he looked on. Before he left he turned and said, 'Oh, by the way, Ahmed will be doing his inspection after the weekend, so make sure you leave the flat clean.'

'No problem,' I smiled.

When we left the bank we went straight back to our 'suitably furnished accommodation' with the dirty battered fridge and stained tattered curtains and packed our cases. Early next morning my colleagues Trish, Simon and Lauren took us to the airport. Lauren hugged us and said, 'Forget all this crap. But don't forget us. And all our good times.'

'Enjoy Brazil, and the wedding,' said Simon. 'I wish you could have stayed here for ours.'

Trish said, 'I'll be leaving this place soon myself. I wouldn't want to stay here with you gone. I'll find myself a place in the world where there are four seasons, and things to look forward to.'

The plane rose into the sky. Between streaks of cloud I glimpsed miles and miles and miles and miles of desert. But we were on our way home and we were smiling.

# TWENTY

# Return to Brazil

At the airport in Uberlândia our friends were waiting: Camacho, David, Lilia, Marilia and Sebastião, and their children, Anna Carolina and Eduardo. These two were no longer the boisterous six-year-olds that Rebecca had referred to in exasperation as 'the shit-heads', but tall, composed, gorgeous 15-year-olds. Our friends folded us into their arms.

David and Lilia's house had not changed at all in nine years and time telescoped to the point where I wouldn't have been at all surprised to see Rebecca and Betsy burst through the door, shrieking with laughter about the macho men on the farm who thought they knew how to ride. The door opened, but only Betsy walked through. Looking at our friends' faces I knew they too saw a Rebecca-shaped space beside her.

Lilia's spinning wheel sat in the same corner. David's books still covered the table in his library. The boxer puppy that Rebecca had loved, creaked up the steps on her nine-year-old legs, accompanied by a puppy of her own.

David and Lilia's new school was an old house in the historic part of the city. They'd bought and renovated it, with meticulous attention to detail, with the proceeds from the sale of their farm nine months ago. They showed us photographs of a run-down house surrounded by other buildings in the same derelict state. It was hard to believe the house was the same one we were admiring now in its little garden full of flowers and trees. David described, with great pride, how neglected the neighbourhood had been when they'd first bought the building and how people stopped by to ask the names of the plants they saw going into the garden.

'You see that boutique over the road? Well, that used to be a rat-infested hovel.

That café next door was the same. People saw what we were doing and they saw the potential in buying these places and restoring them. The whole neighbourhood is on the up. And they've all got gardens. That's something you rarely see here. The whole area is regenerating.'

He ran public speaking and English language courses at the school. On top of that he was still working at the university. Lilia had retired from her job as Linguistics Professor and now taught some of the courses here at the school. She had also started studying music and singing.

We told them how amazed we were at their seemingly unending supply of energy and enthusiasm for new projects. However, I couldn't believe they'd really sold the farm after all their hard work and all their hopes for the riding school. It had been a difficult decision, David agreed, but they'd been fighting a losing battle for years. Every time he'd gone there something had been stolen. Even the horse picture Rebecca had painted, which he'd given pride of place to in the riding school library, had been taken. In addition, the council wouldn't give them any funds towards the Riding for the Disabled School and they were losing money. The last straw was when the farmer next door started a factory for stripping lead from batteries.

'Rebecca always intended to come back,' I said. 'She wanted to work on the farm again. She would have been so sad to think it was no longer part of your life.'

'Betsy feels the same,' Lilia said. 'She still hasn't gotten over it.'

They showed us the plot of land next door that they'd bought for Betsy. When she qualified as a physiotherapist they'd build her a clinic there. First she'd go to the USA to complete her Master's degree. There'd been a bit of a delay while her boyfriend's visa was being processed. Gorgeous, grown-up Betsy, no longer the teenager who didn't like studying. A fully-fledged adult.

As we stood talking on the verandah of the school we saw Terezinha, our Portuguese teacher, walk down the street. She saw us at the same moment and stopped and stared. She threw up her hands and shrieked and ran across the road to where we stood. More hugs and kisses and tears. She immediately began to talk about Rebecca. She couldn't believe it, when Lilia told her! Oh, *meu Deus*! She'd prayed so much. Oh, meu Deus, how did we cope? It was not bearable. It was not imaginable. Rebecca was so *beautiful*. So *talented*. She'd never forgotten her. The way she could *draw*. The way she *laughed*. We must come to her house on Thursday. This was unbelievable that we were here in Uberlândia. This was not possible that at this very moment she'd seen us when just this very morning she'd been thinking of us. She still had the drawing Rebecca had given her as a gift at the end of her last Portuguese lesson. She'd get it out and show it to us on Thursday.

I asked David if he'd take us to see the farm. He said he'd get Betsy to take us as he couldn't bear to see any changes that might be going on there now. On the way to the farm Betsy described her shock when she found out it had been sold. It had happened while she was in the USA. She was so angry, she said, though she could understand the reasons behind it, but if it had been up to her, she wouldn't have sold it.

'And Dad doesn't even want to see it now because it would devastate him to see what they've done. The farm and the riding school were his dream. And he *sold* it!'

'We can't live in the past, Betsy,' Chris said. 'It's good they've moved on.'

'I know. But *still*.'

In the years between us leaving Brazil and Rebecca's death they'd sent us many newspaper clippings and updates about the new buildings on the farm and the progress of the riding school. Now we were travelling back down the red dirt road with Betsy and time was rapidly reversing. There was the bush where Rebecca had seen her first wild snake. There was the tree with the branch lying near the baked red earth where Rebecca and Bruno had stood for a photograph on our last day at the farm.

We pulled up by the old stables and got out of the car. The roof over the horse stalls had fallen in and scattered over the ground. An old saddle lay on a beam, covered in bird droppings. I remembered Fabiano on his weekend visit trying to help Rebecca saddle the horse and her elbowing him out of the way in irritation.

'*Are all New Zealand girls like her – so … so … so …?*'

'Stroppy?' Chris suggested.

'*No no. Independent?*'

We walked along the track past the empty chicken house towards the lake, past the place I'd taken a photo of her riding Cristiane with Beija-Flor trotting alongside and the gander waddling behind.

'She never walked anywhere, did she?' Betsy said. 'She always ran. And jumped over gates. That's what I remember. And the number of times she got thrown off the horses and got straight back on.' She laughed. 'You never knew about the falls, did you?'

I shook my head.

'Just as well!'

There was the little white house where Waltersede had lived with his parrot Rosa.

We walked past the goat house, the mango trees and the enormous red termite mounds. I couldn't wait to see the wooden house by the lake where Rebecca had stayed overnight with Betsy, where we'd picnicked with Fabiano and Bruno and sung songs on the verandah in the rain. We opened the blue gate and walked down the track to the house.

The house had gone.

In its place were foundations, cement mixers, piles of bricks.

Betsy sucked in her breath. 'Oh, *no*! It's just as well Dad didn't come. If he saw this …'

We stood in stunned silence.

Chris started talking about the photo we'd taken of a bird's nest at the side of the old house. 'It had a flower sticking out of it,' he said. 'Rebecca loved it. She said it looked as though the bird had decorated it.'

Betsy had tears in her eyes. Would we please send her a copy of that photo?

I asked her if she remembered the enormous black hairy spider they'd seen the night they stayed in the old house.

She did.

'Rebecca was very impressed with that spider,' I laughed.

Betsy laughed too, but tears splashed onto her cheeks.

I left Chris and Betsy by the lake and crossed the dam to the other side. Sitting in the grass, with closed eyes, I could no longer see their faraway figures staring in dismay at the new house. I could see Rebecca running across the dam after Bruno with handfuls of mud, shrieking with laughter.

The horses coming down to the water to drink.

Rebecca on Cristiane, followed by Beija-Flor, the dogs and the gander.

Lilia preparing the barbecue.

Chris and David working on the new trail.

'*Ajuda!*' screeched Rosa.

I sat in the long grass with my knees drawn up to my chin and opened my eyes. Swallowtails skimmed the surface of the water.

Betsy led us through the track that Chris and Rebecca had helped cut out of the bush. David had often written to Rebecca about how the track had developed and thanked her for her suggestions on how it should be formed. As we drove back up the dirt road, away from the farm, I looked back to the paddock where Rebecca had said goodbye to Cristiane, her face buried in the horse's mane.

When we returned to their house in the city David asked what changes there were. Betsy told him the house had gone.

'*Gone*? You mean they've pulled it *down*?'

Betsy nodded.

David lowered his head to his chest.

I gave them a CD of 'The Red Bandanna', which I'd written for National Radio.

'It's all in there,' I said. 'Even Rosa and the goat!'


In the evening Sebastião picked us up and took us to Araguari. We went to the school where I'd taught Marilia's teachers, Eliane and Katrina. Marilia had written to me when Eliane died of breast cancer and told me now that Katrina was fulfilling her dream of living and working in the States. Magna, Marilia's sister, ran down the stairs at the sound of our voices, and opened her arms wide. Her baby was now eight, she told us. And did we know she had another child?

'Of course they know,' laughed Sebastião. 'Is always a baby in our family. You remember saying that, Sandra?'

I did. I remembered everything.

Next day we walked around Araguari. To our delight we were able to buy a CD of Calvino's songs. Eduardo, the little brat who'd so sorely tried Rebecca's patience, politely answered our questions and helped us buy our tickets to Belo Horizonte. Rebecca wouldn't have believed the change in him.

We took the bus back to Uberlândia in the evening. How I'd loved the bus rides after I'd finished teaching at Marilia's school and I wanted to see once again one of those fabulous sunsets. However, it was winter now, so darkness fell early. Instead, we sat back and let the cadences of the Portuguese language rise and fall about our ears and we smiled at the familiarity and comfort of the sound.

Camacho met us at the bus station in Uberlândia and took us to his house where we met Stela and their daughters, Tatiana and Gabriella, who were now 20 and 16. They were fascinated with our tales of life in Oman, particularly the restrictions on girls and women. I asked Camacho if he could arrange for us to go to Marilena's house. He said he would ring the tenant.

Marilena's house was being rented by an artist. He was dying of cancer, but gave permission for us to go to see the house. He hoped we wouldn't mind, but he wouldn't come down to greet us as he was going through a bad patch. However, we were welcome to wander through the gardens and downstairs rooms and take as long as we liked.

Marilena's furniture and paintings were gone, but it was easy to reconstruct them as we wandered from room to room. There was Rebecca doing her correspondence school work in her bedroom, papers all over the floor; the study where she and Bruno played computer games; the verandah where we lay in hammocks reading books; Seu Pedro hoicking and spitting and pointing out flowers to us and teaching us their names.

There was the mango tree. The long branch with the shape of an impaled woman that I'd seen out of our bedroom window had gone. Later, when we met up with Marilena in Washington, she told me Marlí hadn't liked the branch and she'd sawn it off when she moved into the house after Marilena's departure to the USA. I looked for the owl, but perhaps he'd died.

Marilena's voice: '*I'm getting old. Old and lonely. Soon it will be too late for me to meet anyone.*'

And Bia's voice: '*Don't worry. We'll live here forever like two old maids. And Sandra and Chris and Rebecca, you must come back. I can't imagine this house without you.*'

Five years ago Marilena had married Bernard here in her garden. Bia was living in Recife. Seu Pedro and Dona Antonia worked for someone else now. The dogs and geese were gone. The hammocks were gone. The table where I'd worked every morning was gone. The seats where Marilena and Bia sang and played their guitars on warm evenings were still there. From the garden I looked in at Rebecca's bedroom through the open shutters. How casual I'd been about her presence then.

I returned from my explorations to where Chris and Camacho were waiting on the verandah. We stood in silence, weeping.

Camacho dropped us off in town and we walked past the apartment where we'd lived when we'd first arrived in Uberlândia. I wondered about Reuben. Lilia had told us he'd gone to university and finished his degree in computer science. I hoped he'd achieved his dream of building a house on the land he'd bought.

We crossed the road to buy an ice cream from the shop we used to go to every evening, where the owner had taught us the names of the flavours. A different man was behind the counter now. The tiny blue church that looked like a music box was still there and all the old buildings that we remembered. We wandered further and sat under the *sibipiruna* tree, a huge ancient tree outside a bar where we used to go with Marilena.

Was.

Were.

Did.

Used to.

We walked to Terezinha's house. On the way Chris said it felt as though we were on our way for another lesson and he could feel a headache coming on because he hadn't done his homework. I told Terezinha and she roared with laughter. With her limited English and our rusty Portuguese we were able to convey to her what had happened to Rebecca. I was glad so many people wanted to know and were not afraid to ask.

Terezinha showed us the drawing of a hummingbird that Rebecca had given her. 'Sandra, Chris, some people say it's God's will,' she said. 'But me – I no believe that.'

I nodded and traced the outline of the *beija-flor* with my finger.

In the evening sulphurous yellow clouds billowed like sails and lightning split the sky. Rolls of thunder announced the beginning of the rainy season. Chris went out for a meal with Camacho and some people from the university. Lilia and I settled at the kitchen table. She said when they'd first heard about Rebecca being diagnosed with cancer they couldn't believe it and they'd sat at this table and cried. We cried now, while the rain lashed down in diagonal streaks and thunder rattled the walls.

I told her we were going to Fabiano's wedding.

'He decided to get married to Roberta while we were in Brazil, so we could be there.'

Lilia put her hand over mine.

Camacho and Sebastião called in to say goodbye. The days in Uberlândia with these good, kind people and our revisiting the places that had meant so much to us and to Rebecca had been tremendously hard, but something we both needed to do. I was only sad that we couldn't see Marlí as she was living in another city.

As we got on the plane Chris asked me if I regretted returning to Brazil.

'No. No regrets. Do you regret spending the year in Oman instead of Brazil?'

'In some ways. But overall … probably not.'

Fabiano was waiting with his sister, Tatiana, at the airport in Belo Horizonte. He opened his arms wide when he saw us.

In Fabiano's apartment, crowded with relatives, Roberta came out of the kitchen. Small with long black hair and large brown eyes, she greeted us in halting English, without smiling. Chris spoke to her in Portuguese and asked her to show him her wedding presents. He succeeded in making her smile, but with me she avoided eye contact.

Fabiano's mother, Cleuza, invited us all over for a meal. When Chris and Fabiano left to pick up some wedding presents, Cleuza brought out her wedding album and showed me her photos. She said she could never bring herself to divorce her husband though they'd been separated for 14 years. I asked if her husband would be at the wedding.

She nodded. 'Fabiano didn't want to invite him, but in the end he agreed to, for my sake.'

In the years to come Fabiano's father became so sick he would have died if Cleuza had not gone back to the farm to take care of him and the family finances. There was a spectacular confrontation in the street between the wife and the mistress and the latter was banished for ever.

For now, however, we knew nothing of the future. Cleuza asked how I felt about attending the wedding.

I told her I was glad Fabiano had found happiness.

She was silent for a moment, then said, 'When he came back from New Zealand his heart was so sick no one could help him. Not me, not his sister. He had no words. Tears, yes. So many tears. But no more singing.'

'And now?'

She reached over and took my hand. 'The day I hear my son sing again, that's when I'll know he's okay.'

The door opened and Chris and Fabiano returned. Cleuza fell silent.

Next morning, Darcy, the mother of Guto, one of my Brazilian students in Christchurch who had known Rebecca, whisked me off to a salon where she'd arranged an appointment for our hair and nails to be done. She insisted on paying. Then we had just enough time to go back to the apartment, get changed and go to the church.

We were part of a group of *padrinhos*, witnesses, and waited outside the large white and gold painted church till Fabiano's mother arrived, 45 minutes late. Cleuza, resplendent in a long red dress, walked up the aisle with Fabiano. Our *padrinho* group followed and sat in front of the 500 guests. Fabiano had make-up on and his hair was gelled. It didn't look like him. When he told me later the make-up was just for the photographs, I heard Rebecca's peals of laughter. The choir that he was a part of started singing 'Climb every mountain' and then Fabiano continued the song by himself, in English. I glanced across at Cleuza. She met my eye and nodded.

When Roberta arrived, Fabiano stepped forward to greet her and take her to the altar. The priest, who was also Roberta's godfather, announced that Sandra and Chris, Fabiano's good friends, had come all the way from New Zealand to attend the wedding, then he repeated the same in English and welcomed us 'with joy and happiness'.

The reception was held on the top floor of a nightclub and a band played live music. The control on the sound system had broken and the volume was at head-shattering level. It was impossible to hear any conversation so we moved to the balcony outside.

'Are you okay?' Chris asked.

'Yes. But it would be good to leave soon.'

As we turned to go we walked into Roberta. Her eyes clouded over when she saw me. Without thinking, I reached up and stroked her face. She smiled all the way to her eyes.

After only one night away, Fabiano and Roberta spent the next few days travelling to historic cities in Minas Gerais with us, Darcy and Darcy's sister. Darcy had found us a big old house to stay in and brought mountains of blankets and pillows and food. A strange honeymoon for Roberta, but it gave us the opportunity to get to know her and to love her.

The night before we left Brazil, we went to the wedding of Marilia and Sebastião's nephew, Frederiko, who had ridden in the tractor with Rebecca on Valerio's farm. When we got to the church, Frederiko, Angelo and Leonardo greeted us. They looked exactly as they had eight years before. Leonardo introduced us to his girlfriend in English, 'Here are Rebecca's mother and father.'

All Marilia's family was there with the babies we'd known, now all grown up. I'd been looking forward to seeing Evalbe again, but he wasn't able to attend. At the end of the service, as Andrea Bocelli's 'Time to Say Goodbye' filled the church, I hoped nobody noticed my tears.

We hoped to stay long enough at the reception to meet Valerio, who was going to arrive later, but finally fatigue and the fact we had to go to the airport early next morning, forced us to leave early. Sebastião put his arms around us as we left the reception. His eyes were wet.

Next morning, we said a subdued goodbye to everyone and to Brazil and flew to Washington to see Marilena.

At the baggage carousel I heard an excited shriek. We turned to see Marilena with her arms open wide and Bernard smiling beside her.

In the next few days, in her beautiful house, and exploring Washington DC, we talked and talked and talked. And cried together. She asked me to tell her how Rebecca died.

Before we left I asked her if she was happy.

Well, she said, she was happy with Bernard, but she missed her busy life in Brazil. Here, she couldn't find a permanent job. Americans classified her as a Latino and assumed she wasn't educated or capable. So she'd become a 'Stepford Wife', she laughed, and showed me the hand-painted tiles she'd made for the bathroom. Now that Bruno and Andréia were expecting their first baby, it would be even harder for her not to be living in Brazil. They were waiting for the results of the scan. She was hoping it would be a girl.

And Bruno? Was he happy?

She believed he was.

# TWENTY-ONE

# But she's still dead

Susannah picked us up at the airport. She was all soft skin, glossy brown hair and wide smiles. Oh how I'd missed her!

The familiar roads leading to home. The disconnected feeling of having been away for a long time. Past and present melding. So many faces, so much conversation, so many kindnesses, so many adventures. Was it good to be home? Perhaps it would be, but for now I was still on the outside of that fabric.

When we got home I went straight to Rebecca's bedroom. Although Sue had been living in the house for the past year with her two children, it was exactly as we'd left it. Chris came in behind me.

'She's still dead,' I wept.

'Yes,' he said. 'She is.'

Next morning I opened an email from Trish relating how the accountant of the language school in Muscat had vented his considerable fury when he found out I'd slipped through his fingers. He told her he wouldn't pay her final month's salary. He'd listed her as an absconder. If she attempted to leave Oman to go on her planned holiday to Venice she'd be arrested. She went to the British Embassy which informed him otherwise. A fortnight after that she left the company and the country to fly to a new job. The accountant's last petty act of revenge was to withhold her salary till she was at the check-in counter at the airport, where she was handed an envelope containing her salary in cash. She counted it out to check that every cent had been paid. Lauren and Simon were refused the letter of release they needed to take up a lucrative job offer with another company in Oman at the end of their contract, so they would leave the country to work in Indonesia.

The next email was from the school demanding the immediate return of my Labour Card. The Ministry of Manpower wouldn't allow the company to employ another teacher until the Labour Card was returned, the manager fumed. Leaving a week early like that was a breach of my contract that would make it difficult to convince the company to pay other teachers at the end of their contracts. I should be mindful of my responsibility to them and to the school, especially considering all the time and support that had been devoted to my contractual issues. I must, therefore, return the Labour Card without further delay.

Various responses ran through my mind, especially 'No problem. I'll get back to you, *inshallah*.' In the end I wrote a few lines pointing out that as the company had broken its contract with me in the non-payment of my return airfare, I had no interest whatsoever in any inconvenience my departure had caused. And left it at that.

Then I wrote a reply to my student Amal's email. I told her I was sure she'd do well in Australia. Yes, I missed her too, and all the other students. And yes, we'd had a wonderful time visiting our friends in Brazil and the USA. And yes, oh yes, we were happy to be home.

We took down Rebecca's posters and calendars and repainted the walls. We moved her single bed into the spare room and bought a new double bed. I moved her big oak desk into my study. A few weeks later we packed her clothes in a box and put them into the attic. I laid my sheepskin coat on top before we closed the lid of the box. Susannah had asked me never to throw that coat out. It reminded her of her childhood, she said, when the world felt safe.

Over the following weeks we worked in the overgrown garden and paddocks till they were beautiful again. We arranged for the house to be repainted, and bought new curtains and furniture. We visited friends and marvelled at the green beauty of New Zealand. We went back to our jobs. I started a Master's degree in Creative Writing. The experience of living in Oman had filled me with creative energy and the MLitt gave me a framework to hang my stories on.

I dreamt of Rebecca running towards me and hugging me. I told her it had been such a long time. She said she was working with children now. I laughed, 'What, *you*? Working with *children*? How come?' She said she'd seen an ad and answered it. 'It's like a university,' she said. In another dream she came running and skipping towards me. She held my hand and wanted to talk. She told me she was under specialist care and had to follow a special diet. She looked well and vibrant. I was amazed as the last time I'd seen her she was on the point of death. In the dream I rang The Compassionate Friends and they listened to my story. I realised Rebecca was living independently and was following proper medical advice to get well. I could stop worrying. She knew what to do and was doing it. A child-version of Rebecca heard me talking to TCF and asked if Rebecca was really well. I said, 'She's not out of the woods yet, but she's making progress.' The adult Rebecca told me she lived in a flat and had just taken her flatmate to hospital. That's why she'd decided to come and visit me to let me know she was okay.

These dreams have continued ever since. One was a dream of Rebecca at age five. She sat on my knee, sucking her thumb and drifting off to sleep. I stroked her cheek, marvelling at her. Susannah as an adult stood watching us, smiling. When Rebecca awoke I covered her face in kisses. Someone asked her if the holidays were now over. She said, 'Yes, they're full of over.' I began to wake up, struggling to remind myself of Susannah's and Benjamin's ages. Then I remembered Rebecca was dead. However, unlike all previous such remembrances, which jarred me to full consciousness, the realisation was wrapped inside the feeling of the dream. As I became fully awake, the words of a song I'd recently heard played in my head. *Remember me and smile, I'm in your heart forever … for the love we shared … until we're together again.*

Mark's sister, Melanie, had been looking after Jade and Red. I found a buyer for Jade and Melanie kept Red. Susannah enrolled us both in spinning classes and we bought three alpacas and put them in the empty paddocks. We spun their fleece, sitting on the verandah overlooking the mountains.

I missed riding the horses so much that Chris suggested we buy bikes so we could cycle around the country roads where we lived. This was never as exciting as riding horses on the riverbeds, but it helped fill the gap. Rebecca's huntaway, Scrappy, looked forward to these rides and he became a lot trimmer and fitter racing alongside us. We practised going longer and longer distances, until three years later we were eventually fit enough to ride the 150-kilometre Rail Trail in Central Otago. Gradually, in this way, I wove myself back into my life in New Zealand and it felt the right place to be.

In the months following our return, I searched for the little china cat that Rebecca had always kept stuck on the head of her bed. We'd bought it for her when she was small and it had accompanied her to Brazil and back. As winter turned to spring and spring turned to summer and summer turned to autumn my need to find this cat became more urgent. I searched in every cupboard and every corner and felt desolate that it had gone missing. I couldn't think what could have happened to it or even the last time I'd seen it.

On 6 April the morning of the third anniversary, I was hoeing the flower bed near Rebecca's bedroom window, once again thinking of the little cat and feeling sad that it had been lost. The hoe struck something hard in the soil. *A stone*, I thought, and picked it up. It was the china cat.

On 1 April, four years to the day when Fabiano had said goodbye to Rebecca at Christchurch Airport, Chris and I were back in the same airport waiting for him, Roberta and their one-year-old son, Iago. This time it was we who were waiting with our arms open wide.

As Roberta walked through the front door of our house, she stopped and looked around. 'Oh, I looking forward so long time to come here. To see and know what Fabiano have seen and know.'

Fabiano put his bags down and picked up Sing and Song, Rebecca's cats. A fantail flew through the door. It circled around our heads and perched on a ceiling beam, watching us.

Fabiano's eyes filled with tears.

Roberta looked at me. 'I think she don't mind I am here.'

'No,' I said. 'She doesn't mind.'

Five days later it was the fourth anniversary. At 9.30pm Roberta took Iago and went to bed, leaving Chris and me with Fabiano. We lit a candle and sat quietly, watching the flickering flame.

'I didn't know how I'd feel, coming back this time,' Fabiano said. 'But I really wanted Roberta and Iago to be part of it, whatever happened. As she told you herself, to see and to know what I see and know. And it feels so strange. It's not just the empty spaces here in the house, it's everywhere I go and everywhere I look.'

Chris and I nodded.

'I wish I could've stayed till the end,' Fabiano said. 'I should've cancelled my ticket and the new job and stayed with her.'

'She couldn't leave till you did,' Chris said.

Fabiano let out a long, slow breath.

LOSING A DAUGHTER TO CANCER

I told him of the ways in which Rebecca had given us gifts on each anniversary. 'This time her gift is your being here with us now. Did you know when you booked your ticket that you'd arrive on the exact day you departed four years ago?'

'Not at first. But when I realised … *oh!*'

The baby was asleep. Fabiano and Chris were busy downloading music in Chris's study. Roberta sat beside Susannah at the table, working on a needle-felted teddy bear that Susannah was teaching her how to make.

'The time has gone so fast,' Susannah said. 'I wish you could stay longer than just one month.'

Roberta's large dark eyes sparkled. 'This feel like my home. Except for my mother I no want to return to Brazil. Maybe one day we can come back to live here. Fabiano he always want this. On our first date he bring photos he take in New Zealand and he tell me that even though Rebecca no want him he still will live there because you are like his family.'

Susannah asked if it would be difficult for her to uproot to New Zealand now she had a baby.

Roberta shook her head. 'Iago he is a baby who is so easy for anything.' She paused, searching for words. 'Well, I want to tell you something. Just three weeks after my wedding I know I am pregnant. I was no prepare for such a thing. I cry and cry. Then my mother she tell me I should talk to my baby in my belly so I can know him and he won't feel strange for me. I talk to him for nine months. But,' she hesitated again, 'I have say this to no one before, not even Fabiano. Every time I talk to my child, I no talking to the baby inside my body. My feeling is I talking to a man who standing by my side. A much older, wiser man than me.'

Susannah glanced at me.

'I feel so scared for this responsibility,' Roberta went on. 'When my baby is born, I can no see him like a baby. I do not want this responsibility. I am so afraid. Then, after 50 days I understand he have chose me for his mother. He want me take care him like a baby, not like a man. So then, I decide I have to be his mother. And he have to be my baby.'

Returning from a trip to town we found a wooden plaque engraved with our surname propped up against the front door. That evening Bart rang to ask if we'd got it. When he found we weren't at home he'd left the plaque he'd made for us and gone down to the river to try to find the bridge where he, Grant and Natasha and Rebecca had scratched their initials, eight years ago. To his great disappointment he couldn't find the bridge. I told him Chris and I would go down on our bikes and search for it.

A few days later he arrived with Natasha and we all, Fabiano, Roberta and Iago, drove down to the river where we showed them where the bridge had been stored. It was in two parts now and covered in weeds. We searched every inch of the old bridge, but could find no trace of their initials. Bart didn't want to give up. 'It was here, I'm sure of it,' he said, but in the end he agreed that the wooden planks were so scratched and weathered it was impossible to make out anything resembling their initials.

# TWENTY-TWO

# Celebration

Autumn turned to winter. One morning in June we woke to a dense, heavy silence and looked out the window to see snow had fallen in the night. The trees and plants in the garden had shape-shifted under a thick, white blanket. The roads were blocked and the electricity and phone were cut off. We'd seen nothing like this in all the years we'd lived in New Zealand. Susannah took photos. A tractor was the only vehicle that moved along the road that day. Susannah wouldn't be able to drive home till the roads were cleared, which, by the look of things, would be several days, so none of us would be able to get to work. We pulled out photo albums to find pictures of Susannah making a snowman at my mother's house in England when she was 11. We spent the day going through all the albums, Susannah's, Benjamin's, Rebecca's, Chris's, mine, my parents', Chris's parents'. And we told each other what we remembered.

'Do you remember when Rebecca saw snow in England for the first time?' said Chris. 'She thought it was ice cream and launched herself into it.'

We all laughed out loud and Chris talked about the sleds his father used to make him every Christmas when he was a child and I told Susannah how strange it felt having Christmas in the summer when we first came to New Zealand.

In the evening we piled on coats, hats and scarves and plodded along the road in the deep tracks the tractor had made.

'It looks like a different country,' Susannah said.

'They look like those turtle tracks in Oman,' Chris and I said simultaneously.

The sun had almost disappeared behind the mountains and purple shadows lay across the snow. I thought of all the tulips and daffodils and snowdrops and bluebells in the gardens we passed, dormant now in the dark earth.

We reached the top of the road and turned the corner to see the moon. A giant peach in a blueberry sky. Susannah took more photographs.

'Oh Mum,' she breathed, 'it's so beautiful it makes you want to cry.'

Chris put his arm around her.

When Rebecca died I told Susannah that I was worried he didn't cry. She said, 'His kind of crying is like bleeding internally. Nothing seems to be happening on the outside. The tears are all deep inside. It's the same with me.'

When Rebecca died Benjamin didn't have enough words to describe his anger with God. So he stopped writing songs and playing his music and packed his guitar and keyboard away in a cupboard.

After the snowstorm he rang me from Wellington to say a friend had sent him a poem and he thought he could write some music for it. He took his guitar and keyboard out of the cupboard. He would email me the song when he'd finished it, but it would sound better on the piano than the keyboard. Could I have the piano tuned before his next visit to Christchurch?

At the end of the year Chris and I started going to tango lessons. One day while we were gardening he put a tango CD in the car and turned the volume up loud. We did the tango up and down the drive in our gardening boots and danced barefoot on the lawn. We collapsed laughing in each other's arms.

'Who'd have thought?' we said.

In the summer, Natasha and Bart came to visit. Natasha brought a bunch of tightly furled roses from her garden and pointed to a dark pink one.

'It's called Best Friend,' she said. 'I planted it when we bought the new house.'

She gave us a photo of Rebecca at her sister's wedding. Natasha's sister, now divorced, had found the photo while clearing out the garage.

Bart laughed when he saw the photo. 'It's the first one I've ever seen of Becks wearing a dress and smiling at the same time!' he said. And we all laughed with him. He brought out an album of his photos of the old car. He'd got together with Grant and they'd gone through all their photos to see if they could identify that part of the bridge where they'd scratched their initials. But, no joy, he said. Anyway, he'd leave the album with us to look at and he'd pick it up on his next visit.

Natasha told us that on a recent visit to a relative in hospital the 'best friend' necklace that Rebecca had given her suddenly snapped and fell to the ground. 'I remembered then that she told me she never wanted to go back to that hospital,' she said. 'So I picked up the chain and took it back to my car and put it in the glove box.'

As we were saying goodbye to Natasha and Bart six hours later, I pointed to the vase of roses to say thank you once again. The other roses were still tightly furled, but the Best Friend rose had fully opened.

'Weird, eh?' said Bart.


Susannah decided not to have children. Benjamin said he wanted no more. On their 10th wedding anniversary, Benjamin and Dee separated. I mourned the loss of all those grandchildren I'd once hoped for. I dreamt I had a dead baby. When everyone arrived for her funeral I brought her out to show them. Their eyes were dark with horror as I laid her on a table and washed and dressed her and wrapped her up in a shawl.

'You should have buried it before now!' someone said.

'She's a *girl*,' I said. 'Not an *it*. She has a name. She's a human being and that's how I'm going to bury her.'

Susannah dreamt that Rebecca showed her a little boy whom, she realised, was the son Susannah might have had, but the opportunity for bringing him into the world had been lost. 'He was lovely. Very gentle and sensitive,' she wept. 'But I know that if I did bring him here, something terrible would happen to him and I couldn't face that much pain.'

A colleague spoke to me of the birth of her premature baby. She held the child for two hours till she died. She spoke of how her milk came in two days later. How sometimes she patted her stomach and was surprised to find no bump. 'But the worst thing was seeing the scan,' she said. 'There was just a dark space where the baby should have been.'

That night I dreamt I was in a shop looking at clothes. I was pleased to see a section for baby clothes and I looked at them to buy something for Rebecca. Then I remembered she was dead and realised Benjamin had died too. I was left with one child. I looked in a cupboard and saw all the quilts my children had had on their cots when they were babies. I found myself on a hill trying to breathe. Chris came towards me and saw the look on my face. As he held me my breathing turned into wailing. I woke up feeling scraped hollow.


In September 2008 Benjamin said he was coming home for my birthday. I hadn't celebrated this day since 2001 when Rebecca had gone into hospital with peritonitis. Now I felt like cooking a lovely meal and celebrating the life we had, with our two beautiful adult children.

Susannah made her usual trip out to the paddocks to see the three alpacas and the two Boer goats we'd reared since last Christmas. Blair, our Angora, had died at age nine, five months before we got them. When she returned to the house she said, 'All those animals make the paddocks happy again.'

As we clinked our glasses of wine at dinner, Susannah said that while she was driving over the ford towards our house, she had an impression of Rebecca galloping on her horse alongside the car.

'It was like she was racing me. I even turned to look at her, but of course there was no one there. Nevertheless, I was certain she turned and smiled at me. I feel she's really excited, Mum. She's really happy that we're all here together. That we're celebrating this day.'

*Hold this moment.*

*Hold it.*

*Breathe it into my bones.*

# Bibliography

Addison, S. (2001), *Mother Lode: Stories of home life and home death*. St Lucia, Australia: University of Queensland Press

Allende, I. (1995), *Paula*. London: Flamingo

Allende, I. (2008), *The Sum of Our Days*. London: HarperCollins

Anderson, R. (1988), 'Channelling', *Parapsychology Review*, September–October, pp. 4–9

Anon (2007), 'An interview with Jenny Downham', *New York Times*: www.nytimes.com/2007/10/14/books/review/interview-downham.html?ref=review (accessed Feb 2011)

Anon (2001), 'The age of creative nonfiction', *Nidus* (Fall): www.pitt.edu/-nidus/archives/fall2001/rt1.html (accessed September 2007)

Arbuckle, N. W. & B. de Vries (1995), 'The long-term effects of later life spousal and parental bereavement on personal functioning', *Gerontologist 35*, pp. 637–47

Averill, J. R. (1968), 'Grief: Its nature and significance', *Psychological Bulletin 70*, pp. 721–48

Barrett, D. (1991–1992), 'Through a glass darkly: Images of the dead in dreams', *Omega 24* (2), pp. 97–106

Bates, B. C. & Stanley, A. (1984), 'What drowning feels like', *British Medical Journal 2*, pp. 823–24

Bernstein, J. R. (1997), *When the Bough Breaks*. Kansas City: Andrews McMeel Publishing

Betty, S. (2006), 'Are they hallucinations or are they real? The spirituality of deathbed and near-death visions', *Omega 53* (1–2), pp. 37–49

Birch, J. M. et al (2003), 'Incidence of malignant disease by morphological type, in young persons aged 12–24 years in England (1979–1997)', *European Journal of Cancer 39* (18)

Blackmore, S. (1993), *Dying to Live: Science and near-death experiences*. London: HarperCollins

Blank, J. W. (1998), *The Death of an Adult Child*. Amityville, New York: Baywood Publishing Co. Inc.

Bolton, G. (2000), 'Opening the word hoard', *Medical Humanities 26*, pp. 55–57

Bolton, G. et al (2003), 'Who's speaking?', *Journal of Medical Ethics 29* (2), p. 97

Bond, S. (2006), Review, *API Review of Books 44*: www.api-network.com/cgi-bin/reviews/jrbview.cgi?n=0702231916 (accessed 14 July 2007)

Bone, P. (2007), *Bad Hair Days*. Melbourne: Melbourne University Press

Bonnano, G. et al (1995), 'When avoiding unpleasant emotions might not be such a bad thing', *Journal of Personality and Social Psychology 69* (5), pp. 975–89

Bowlby, J. (1961), 'Process of mourning', *International Journal of Psycho-Analysis 42*, pp. 317–40

Bowlby, J. & Parkes, C. M. (1970), 'Separation and loss within the family', in Anthony, E. J. (ed.) *The Child in His Family*, New York: Wiley, pp. 197–216

Bowlby, J. (1980), *Attachment and Loss: Vol 3. Loss: Sadness and depression*. New York: Basic Books

Brailsford, B. (1999), *Wisdom of the Four Winds*. Christchurch: Stoneprint Press

Brien, D. L. (2001), 'Creative nonfiction 2: A virtual conversation with Michael Steinberg', *Text 5* (1)

Cacace, M. F. & E. Williamson (1996), 'Grieving the death of an adult child', *Journal of Gerontological Nursing 22*, pp. 16–22

Cahill, B., R. Skloot & L. Gutkind (2001), 'The age of creative nonfiction', *Nidus*: www.pitt.edu/~nidus/archives/fall2001/rtl.html (accessed 15 September 2007)

Carroll, B. E. (1997), *Spiritualism in Antebellum America*. Bloomington, Indiana: Indiana University Press

Carroll, R. D. (2007), 'Near-death experience', in *The Skeptics Dictionary*: http:/skeptdic.com/nde.html (accessed 8 July 2007)

Causer, G. T. (1997), *Recovering Bodies*. Madison, Wisconsin: University of Wisconsin Press

Clabburn, P. (2007), 'Facing life after losing your son', *BBC News:* http://news.bbc.

co.uk/2/hi/health/7109834.stm (accessed February 2011)

Cohen, S. & B. S. Rabin (1998), 'Psychologic stress, immunity, and cancer', *Journal of the National Cancer Institute 90* (1), pp. 3–4

Cordell, A. & N. Thomas (1990), 'Fathers grieving: Coping with infant death', *Journal of Perinatology 10* (1), pp. 75–80

Cunnane, A. (2007), 'To live outside the law you must be honest', *Booknotes 158*

Daher, D. (2003), *And the Passenger was Death.* New York: Baywood Publishing Co.

Davies, A. M. (2001), 'Death of adolescents: Parental grief and coping strategies', *British Journal of Nursing 10* (20), pp. 1332–42

Davies, D. J. (2002), *Death, Ritual and Belief* (2nd edn). London: Continuum

Davies, O. (1999), *Witchcraft, Magic and Culture.* Manchester: Manchester University Press

Davies, R. (2004), 'New understandings of parental grief: Literature review', *Journal of Advanced Nursing 46* (5), pp. 506–13

Dean, M. et al (2005), 'Parental experiences of adult child death from cancer', *Journal of Palliative Medicine 8* (4), pp. 751–65

Devers, E. & K. M. Robinson (2002), 'The making of a grounded theory: After-death communication', *Death Studies 26* (3), pp. 241–53

Didion, J. (2006), *The Year of Magical Thinking.* London: Fourth Estate

Dillard, A. (1999), 'To fashion a text', in Root, R. & M. Steinberg (eds), *The Fourth Genre: Contemporary writers of/on creative nonfiction.* Boston: Allyn & Bacon, pp. 270–78

Dokken, D. & N. Sydnor-Greenberg (2000), 'Exploring complementary and alternative medicine in pediatrics: Parents and professionals working together for new understanding', *Pediatric Nursing 26* (4), pp. 383–90

Dower, L. (2001), *I Will Remember You.* New York: Scholastic Inc.

Downham, J. (2007), *Before I Die.* Oxford: David Fickling Books

Duder, T. (1998), Foreword, in Gatenby, B., *For the Rest of Our Lives.* Auckland: Reed Books

Dyregrov, K. & A. Dyregrov (2008), *Effective Grief and Bereavement Support.* London: Jessica Kingsley Publishers

Edmond, L. (1991), *Bonfires in the Rain.* Wellington: Bridget Williams Books

Edmond, L. (1992), *The Quick World.* Wellington: Bridget Williams Books

Edwards, E. (2006), *Saving Graces.* New York: Broadway Books

Ekert, H. (1989), *Childhood Cancer: Understanding and coping.* New York: Gordon & Breach Science Publishers

Enright, A. (2007), 'Diary: Disliking the McCanns', *London Review of Books* (4 October): www.lrb.co.uk/v29/n19/enri01_.html (accessed Feb 2011)

Epel, N. (1993), *Writers Dreaming.* New York: Vintage Books

Everett, D. L. (2008), *Don't Sleep, There are Snakes.* London: Profile Books

Finkbeiner, A. (1998), *After the Death of a Child.* Maryland: Johns Hopkins University Press

Fish, W. C. (1986), 'Differences of grief intensity in bereaved parents', in Rando, T. A. (ed.), *Parental Loss of a Child.* Champaign, Illinois: Research Press

Forché, C. & P. Gerard (2001), *Writing Creative Nonfiction.* Cincinnati: Story Press

Fox, D. (2006), 'Light at the end of the tunnel', *New Scientist 192* (2573), pp. 1–4

Frank, A. W. (1995), *The Wounded Storyteller.* Chicago: University of Chicago Press

Freud, S. (1961), 'Mourning and melancholia', in Strachey, J. (ed.), *The Standard Edition of the Complete Psychological Works of Sigmund Freud* (vol. 14). London: Hogarth Press (original work published 1917)

Funerals New Zealand website: www.funeralsnewzealand.co.nz

Garner, H. (2008), *The Spare Room.* Melbourne: Text Publishing Co.

Gatenby, B. (1998), *For the Rest of Our Lives.* Auckland: Reed Books

Gilbert, K. R. (2002), 'Taking a narrative approach to grief research: Finding meaning in stories', *Death Studies 26*, pp. 223–39

Gorer, G. (1965), *Death, Grief and Mourning in Contemporary Britain.* London: Cresset Press

Grant, S. (2005), *Standing on His Own Two Feet: A diary of dying.* London: Jessica Kingsley Publishers

Graves, D. (2009), *Talking with Bereaved People: An approach for structured and sensitive communication.* London: Jessica Kingsley Publishers

Grealy, L. (1996), in Noël, C. *In the Unlikely Event of a Water Landing.* New York: Random House

Greyson, B. (1993), 'Varieties of near-death experience', *Psychiatry 56*, 390–99

Greyson, B. (2000), 'Dissociation in people who have near-death experiences: Out of their bodies or out of their minds?', *The Lancet 355* (9202), pp. 460–63

Greyson, B. (2006), 'Near-death experiences and spirituality', *Zygon 41* (2), pp. 393–414

Griffin, G. M. & D. Tobin (1997), *In the Midst of Life: The Australian response to death*

(2nd edn). Melbourne: Melbourne University Press

Grinyer, A. & C. Thomas (2001), 'Young adults with cancer: The effect of the illness on parents and families', *International Journal of Palliative Nursing 7*, pp. 162–70

Grinyer, A. (2002), *Cancer in Young Adults Through Parents' Eyes*. Buckingham: Open University Press

Grinyer, A. (2003), 'Young adults with cancer: Parents' interactions with health care professionals', *European Journal of Cancer Care 13*, pp. 88–95

Grinyer, A. & C. Thomas (2004), 'The importance of place of death in young adults with terminal cancer', *Mortality 9* (2), pp. 114–31

Grinyer, A. (2006a), 'Caring for a young adult child with cancer: The impact on mothers' health', *Health Social Care in the Community 14* (4), pp. 311–18

Grinyer, A. (2006b), 'Telling the story of illness and death', *Auto/biography 14* (3), pp. 206–22

Gurney, E., F. W. H. Myers & F. Podmore (1886), *Phantasms of the Living*. London: Trubner & Co.

Gutkind, L. (1997), *The Art of Creative Nonfiction*. New York: John Wiley & Sons

Gutkind, L. (n.d.), 'Style and substance', *Creative Nonfiction* (10): http://creativenonfiction.org/thejournal/articles/issue10/10contents.htm (accessed February 2011)

Gutkind, L. (2001), 'Becoming the godfather of creative nonfiction', in Forche, C. & P. Gerard (eds), *Writing Creative Nonfiction*. Cincinnati: Story Press, pp. 170–80

Hampl, P. (1999), 'Memory and imagination', in Root, R. & M. Steinberg (eds), *The Fourth Genre: Contemporary writers of/on creative nonfiction*. Boston: Allyn & Bacon, pp. 297–305

Hannah, L. (n.d.), *Natural Burial Parks*: http//livinglegacies.co.nz/naturalper cent-20burialper cent20parks.htm (accessed February 2009)

Haraldsson, E. (1988–1989), 'Survey of claimed encounters with the dead', *Omega 19* (2), pp. 10–113

Hawes, P. (2005), 'My other life', *Off Campus Magazine: August*: www.massey.ac.nz/~wwexmss/Offcampus/August2005/book_review.html (accessed August 2007)

Hazzard, C., J. Weston & C. Guiterres (1992), 'After a child's death: Factors related to parental bereavement', *Developmental and Behavioural Pediatrics 13*, pp. 24–30

Hedtke, L. (2002), 'Reconstructing the language of death and grief', *Illness, Crisis and Loss 10* (4), pp. 285–93

Hibbert, K. (2007), 'No trace of corn', *Times Online*: http://entertainment.timesonline.co.uk/tol/arts_and_entertainment/books/article1894252.ece (accessed February 2011)

Hoekstra-Weebers, J. E. H. M. et al. (1991), 'A comparison of parental coping styles, following the death of adolescent and pre-adolescent children', *Death Studies* 15, pp. 565–75

Holcroft, M. H. (1989), *The Grieving Time*. Dunedin: John McIndoe

Holloway, J. (1990), 'Bereavement literature: A valuable resource for the bereaved and those who counsel them', *Interdisciplinary Journal of Pastoral Studies 3*, pp. 7–26

Holly, M. L. (1989), 'Reflective writing and the spirit of inquiry', *Cambridge Journal of Education 19*, pp. 71–79

Horacek, J. (1997), 'Amazing grace: The healing effects of near-death experiences on those dying and grieving', *Journal of Near-Death Studies 16* (2), pp. 149–59

Ironside, V. (1996), *You'll Get Over It*. London: Hamish Hamilton

Jackson, P. (2007), 'Coping with death on the web', *BBC News*: http://news.bbc.co.uk/2/hi/6700743.stm (accessed February 2011)

Jones, L. (1993), *Biografi: An Albanian quest*. Wellington: Victoria University Press

Jones, L. (2008), *Biografi: An Albanian quest*. Melbourne: Text Publishing

Jong, E. (1985), 'The life we live and the life we write', *New York Times*: http://www.nytimes.com/books/97/07/20/reviews/8041.html (accessed July 2005)

Joyce, J. (1916), *A Portrait of the Artist as a Young Man*. New York: W. Huebsch

Kaprio, J., M. Koskenvuo & H. Rita (1987), 'Mortality after bereavement: A prospective study of 95 widowed persons', *American Journal of Public Health 77* (3), pp. 283–87

Karr, M. (1995), *The Liars Club*. New York: Viking Press

Kavanaugh, R. J. (1974), *Facing Death*. Baltimore: Penguin

Kellehear, A. (2007), *A Social History of Dying*. Melbourne: Cambridge University Press

Kelly, E. W. (2001), 'Near-death experiences with reports of meeting deceased people', *Death Studies 25*, pp. 229–49

Kelly, E. W., B. Greyson & I. Stevenson (1999–2000), 'The evidence for life after death', *Omega 40* (4), pp. 513–19

Kerouac, J. (1957), *On the Road*. New York: Viking Press

Klass, D. (1993a), 'Solace and immortality: Bereaved parents' continuing bonds with their children', *Death Studies* (17), pp. 342–68

Klass, D. (1993b), 'The inner representation of the dead child and the world views of bereaved parents', *Omega 26*, pp. 255–73

Klass, D., P. Silverman & S. L. Z. Nickman (eds) (1996), *Continuing Bonds: New understandings of grief.* Washington: Taylor & Francis

Klass, D. (1999), *The Spiritual Lives of Bereaved Parents.* Philadelphia: Taylor & Francis

Knapp, R. J. (1986), *Beyond Endurance: When a child dies.* New York: Schoken Books

Kübler-Ross, E. (1970), *On Death and Dying.* London: Tavistock

Kübler-Ross, E. (1975), *Death: The final stage of growth.* New Jersey: Prentice-Hall

Kübler-Ross, E. (1991), *On Life After Death.* Berkeley: Celestial Arts

Kübler-Ross, E. (1997a), *Questions and Answers on Death and Dying.* New York: Touchstone

Kübler-Ross, E. (1997b), *Working it Through.* New York: Touchstone

Laakso, H. & M. Paunonen-Ilmonen (2002), 'Mothers' experience of social support following the death of a child', *Journal of Clinical Nursing 11*, pp. 176–85

LaGrand, L. E. (1997), *After-Death Communication.* Minnesota: Llewellyn Publications

Lang, A. & L. Gottlieb (1993), 'Parental grief reactions and marital intimacy following infant death', *Death Studies 17*, pp. 233–55

Langbauer, W. R. (2000), 'Elephant communication', *Zoo Biology 19*, pp. 425–45

Langley-Lesnik, C. (2008), *Diary of a Cancer Survivor:* http://appendix-cancer.blogspot. com (accessed September 2008)

Larson, T. (2007), *The Memoir and the Memoirist.* Ohio: Swallow Press

Lee, R. L. M. (2008), 'Modernity, mortality and re-enchantment: The death taboo revisited', *Sociology 42* (4), pp. 745–59

Lempert, T., M. Bauer & D. Schmidt (1994), 'Syncope and near-death experience', *The Lancet* (344), pp. 829–30

Lesher, E. L. & K. J. Bergey (1988), 'Bereaved elderly mothers: Changes in health, functional activities, family cohesion, and psychological well-being', *International Journal of Aging and Human Development 26* (2), pp. 381–90

Levav, I. (1982), 'Mortality and psychopathology following the death of an adult child: An epidemiological review', *Journal of Psychiatry and Related Sciences 19* (1), pp. 23–38

Levav, I. et al. (1988), 'An epidemiologic study of mortality among bereaved parents', *New England Journal of Medicine* (319), pp. 457–61

Levine, M. (2004), *First You Die.* USA: Silver Thread Publishers

Lewis, C. S. (1961), *A Grief Observed*. New York: Seabury Press

Littlewood, J. L. et al. (1991), 'Gender differences in parental coping following their child's death', *British Journal of Guidance Counselling 19* (2), pp. 139

Mailer, N. (1979), *The Executioner's Song*. Boston: Little Brown

Marais, E. N. (1973), *The Soul of the Ape*. Harmondsworth: Penguin

Martin, J. & P. Romanowski (2009), *Love Beyond Life: The healing power of after-death communications* (2nd edn). New York: HarperCollins

Marx, R. J. & S. W. Davidson (2003), *Facing the Ultimate Loss*. Fredonia, Canada: Champion Press

Mauro, J. (1992), 'Bright lights, big mystery', *Psychology Today, 54+*.

McAdams, D. P. (1993), *The Stories We Live By: Personal myths and the making of the self*. New York: Guilford Press

McCourt, F. (1996), *Angela's Ashes*. London: HarperCollins

McCourt, F. (1999), *'Tis*. London: Flamingo

McCourt, F. (2005), *Teacher Man*. London: Fourth Estate

McCrum, R. (2007), 'A natural for the Nobel Prize', Christchurch *Press*, 17 October, p. B4

McIntosh, D. N., R. Silver & C. B. Wortman (1993), 'Religion's role in adjustment to a negative life event: Coping with the loss of a child', *Journal of Personality and Social Psychology 65*, pp. 812–21

McNamara, B. (2001), *Fragile Lives: Death, dying and care*. Philadelphia: Open University Press

Miles, M. S. (1985), 'Emotional symptoms and physical health in bereaved parents', *Nursing Research 34*, pp. 76–81

Mitford, J. (1963), *The American Way of Death*. New York: Simon & Schuster

Moody, R. (1975), *Life After Life*. Atlanta: Mockingbird Books

Moody, R. (1993), *Reunions*. New York: Villard Books

Moran, R. (1989), 'Please don't ask me if I'm over it'. *Chicago Tribune*. http://articles. chicagotribune.com/1989-04-27/features/8904070656_1_dear-ann-landers-compassionate-friends-computer-glitch.

Morse, M. L. & P. Perry (1990), *Closer to the Light: Learning from children's near-death experiences*. New York: Villard Books

Moss, C. (1988), *Elephant Memories: 13 years in the life of an elephant family*. New York: William Morris & Co.

Moss, D. M. (2005), 'At the point of death: A case study', *Pastoral Psychology 53* (5), pp. 447–73

Murray, J. A. & D. J. Terry (1999), 'Parental reactions to infant death: The effects of resources and coping strategies', *Journal of Social and Clinical Psychology 18*, pp. 341–69

Nester, D. (2005), 'An interview with Lee Gutkind', *Bookslut*: www.bookslut.com/features/2005_07_005959.php (accessed February 2011)

Nippert, M. (2008), 'The death of funerals', *New Zealand Listener*, 24–30 May: www.listener.co.nz/issue/3550/features/11109/the_death_of-funerals_.html (accessed February 2011)

Noël, C. (2005), *In the Unlikely Event of a Water Landing: A geography of grief*. New York: Authors' Choice Press

Nyatanga, B. (2001), *Why is it so Difficult to Die?* Wiltshire: Quay Books

O'Brien, K. (2008), 'Helen Garner speaks with Kerry O'Brien', *The 7.30 Report*: www.abc.net.au/7.30/content/2007/s2253092.htm (accessed February 2011)

Olff, M. (1999), 'Stress, depression and immunity: The role of defence and coping styles', *Psychiatry Research 85* (1), pp. 7–15

Oliver, R. C. & M. E. Fallat, (1995), 'Traumatic childhood death: How do parents cope?', *Journal of Trauma 39* (2), pp. 303–08

Osis, K. & E. Haraldsson (1977), *At the Hour of Our Death*. New York: Aveon

*Parents' Bereavement Support Group Newsletter* (2004), 'Each in his own way: Children and adolescents living with grief', November

Parkes, C. M. (1986), *Bereavement: Studies of grief in adult life* (2nd edn). London: Tavistock

Parnia, S. (2006), *What Happens When We Die*. Carlsbad, California: Hay House

Pennebaker, J. (2004), *Writing to Heal*. Oakland, California: New Harpinger Publications

Penrod Herman, C. (2001), 'Spiritual needs of dying patients: A qualitative study', *Oncology Nursing Forum 28* (1), pp. 67–72

Rando, T. (1983), 'An investigation of grief and adaptation in parents whose children have died from cancer', *Journal of Pediatric Psychology 8* (1), pp. 3–20

Rando, T. (1984), *Grief, Dying and Death: Clinical interventions for caregivers*. Champaign, Illinois: Research Press

Rando, T. A. (1991), 'Parental adjustment to the loss of a child', in Papadatou, D. & C. Papadatos (eds), *Children and Death*. New York: Hemisphere

Rees, W. D. (1971), The hallucinations of widowhood. *British Medical Journal*, October, pp. 37–41

Riches, G. & P. Dawson (2000), *An Intimate Loneliness: Supporting bereaved parents and siblings.* Buckingham: Open University Press

Riley, L. P. et al (2007), 'Parental grief responses and personal growth following the death of a child', *Death Studies 31* (4), pp. 277–99

Ritchie, G. (1978), *Return from Tomorrow.* Grand Rapids, Michigan: Fleming H. Revell

Robinson, M. (2000), 'Writing well: Health and the power to make images', *Medical Humanities 26*, pp. 79–84

Roorbach, B. (2001), *Contemporary Creative Nonfiction: The art of truth.* New York: Oxford University Press

Root, L. J. & M. Steinberg (1999), *The Fourth Genre.* Boston: Allyn & Bacon

Rosenblatt, P. C. (2000), *Parent Grief: Narratives of loss and relationship.* Philadelphia: Taylor & Francis

Rosof, B. D. (1994), *The Worst Loss.* New York: Henry Holt & Co.

Rossetti, C. (2002), *Snapshots.* Wellington: Steele Roberts

Rubin, S. S. (1989–1990), 'Death of the future? An outcome study of bereaved parents in Israel', *Omega 20*, pp. 323–39

Sabom, M. B. (1982), *Recollections of Death: A medical investigation.* New York: Harper & Row

Sanders, C. M. (1979–1980), 'A comparison of adult bereavement in the death of a spouse, child and parent', *Omega 10*, pp. 303–21

Sanders, C. M. (1989), *Grief; the Mourning After: Dealing with adult bereavement.* Toronto: Wiley & Sons

Schiff, S. (1977), *The Bereaved Parent.* New York: Crown Publishers

Schneider, M. & R. C. Mannell (2006), 'Beacon in the storm: An exploration of the spirituality and faith of parents whose children have cancer'. *Issues in Comprehensive Pediatric Nursing 29*, pp. 3–24

Schnell, L. (2000), 'The language of grief', *Vermont Quarterly* (Fall)

Schwab, R. (1996), 'Gender differences in parental grief', *Death Studies 20*, pp. 103–13

Seguin, M., A. Leage & M. C. Kiely (1995), 'Parental bereavement after suicide and accident: A comparative study', *Suicide and Life Threatening Behaviour* (25), pp. 489–98

Shanfield, S. B., G. A. H. Benjamin & B. J. Swain (1984), 'Parents' reactions to the death of an adult child from cancer', *American Journal of Psychiatry 141*, pp. 1092–94

Sidgewick, H. (1894), 'Report on the census of hallucinations', *Proceedings of the Society for Psychical Research 10*, pp. 25–422

Somanti, M. & August, J. (1997), 'Parental bereavement: Spiritual connections with dead children', *American Journal of Orthopsychiatry 67* (3), pp. 460–69

Spencer, W. (2001), 'To absent friends: Classical spiritualist mediumship and New Age channelling compared and contrasted', *Journal of Contemporary Religion 16* (3)

Spratt, M. L. & D. R. Denney (1991), 'Immune variables, depression and plasma cortisol over time in suddenly bereaved parents', *Journal of Neuropsychiatry and Clinical Neurosciences 3*, pp. 299–306

Staudacher, C. (1987), *Beyond Grief.* Oakland, California: New Harbinger Publications

Stead, C. K. (2008), *Book Self.* Auckland: Auckland University Press

Steiner, R. (1973), *Karmic Relationships.* East Sussex: Rudolph Steiner Press

Stroebe, M. & H. Schut (1999), 'The dual process model of coping with bereavement: Rationale and description', *Death Studies 23* (3), pp. 197–224

Sutherland, C. (1995), *Children of the Light.* New York: Bantam

Tagore, R. (2008), *Stray Birds.* Radford, Virginia: Wilder Publications

Talbot, K. (2002), *What Forever Means after the Death of a Child.* London: Brunner-Routledge

Tatelbaum, J. (1981), *The Courage to Grieve.* London: William Heinemann

Taylor, M. (2003), 'Counselling: The language of grief', *For Peace of Mind* (Summer): http://forpeaceofmind.com.au/vol2/counselling.cfm (accessed February 2011)

The Aware Study (2008), www.mindbodysymposium.com/Human-Consciousness-Project/the-Aware-study (accessed January 2009)

Tonkin, L. (2006), *Getting Through It* (pamphlet), Auckland: Child Cancer Foundation

Van Lommel, P. et al. (2001), 'Near-death experience in survivors of cardiac arrest: A prospective study in the Netherlands', *The Lancet 358*, pp. 2039–45

Wagner, K. (n.d.), 'An interview with the godfather', *Adirondack Review*: http://adiron-dackreview.homestead.com/interviewgutkind.html (accessed February 2011)

Walliss, J. (2001), 'Continuing bonds: Relationship between the living and the dead within contemporary spiritualism', *Mortality 6* (2), pp. 12–145

Walter, T. (1991), 'Modern Death: Taboo or not taboo?' *Sociology 25* (2), pp. 293–310

Walter, T. (1996), 'A new model of grief: Bereavement and biography', *Mortality 1* (1), pp. 7–25

Walter, T. (1999), *On Bereavement: The culture of grief.* Berkshire: Open University Press

Walter, T. (2000), 'Grief narratives: The role of medicine in the policing of grief', *Anthropology & Medicine 7* (1), pp. 97–114

Wattie, N. & R. Chrisinson (eds) (1998), 'Lloyd Jones', in *The Oxford Companion to New Zealand Literature.* Auckland: Oxford University Press

Waugh, E. (1948), *The Loved One.* New York: Dell Publishing Co. Inc.

Welch, D. (2006), 'Staying after school with Frank McCourt': www.powells.com/ authors/mccourt.html (accessed February 2011)

Wills-Brandon, C. (2002), 'Understanding departing visions or deathbed visitation', *Journal of Religion and Psychical Research*, pp. 196–2000

Worden, J. W. (1982), *Grief Counselling and Grief Therapy.* New York: Springer Publishing Co.

Worden, J. W. (1991), *Grief Counselling and Grief Therapy: A handbook for the mental health practitioner* (2nd edn). London: Routledge

Wortman, C. B. & R. C. Silver (1989), 'The myths of coping with loss', *Journal of Consulting and Clinical Psychology 57*, pp. 349–57

Wright, J. & M. Chueng Chung (2001), 'Mastery or mystery? Therapeutic writing: A review of the literature', *British Journal of Guidance 29*, pp. 277–91

Young, H. (2008), 'It is so, so utterly painful': www.stuff.co.nz/print4599463a12855.html

Young, L. (2008), 'I survive on grim stoicism and anti-depressants': www.stuff.co.nz/ print4599463a12855